D0830154

COMMUNICATION INTERVENTION

Birth to Three

Second Edition

COMMUNICATION INTERVENTION
Birth to Three

Second Edition

Louis M. Rossetti, Ph.D.
Speech and Hearing Clinic
Arts and Communication Center
University of Wisconsin—Oshkosh
Oshkosh, Wisconsin

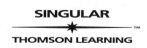

SINGULAR
™
THOMSON LEARNING

Australia   Canada   Mexico· Singapore   Spain   United Kingdom   United States

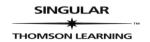

Delmar Staff:

Business Unit Director: Bill Brottmiller

Acquisitions Editor: Marie Linvill

Editorial Assistant: Kristin Banach

Executive Marketing Manager: Dawn Gerrain

Channel Manager: Kathryn Little

Executive Production Manager: Karen Leet

Project Editor: Stacey Prus

Production Editor: Brad Bielawski

Art/Design Coordinator: Jay Purcell

Library of Congress Cataloging-in-Publication Data

Rossetti, Louis Michael.

      Communication intervention : birth to three / by Louis M. Rossetti.—2nd ed.

          p. ; cm.

      Includes bibliographical references and index.

      ISBN 0-7693-0093-6 (soft cover : alk. paper)

      1. Speech Disorders in children.   2. Speech therapy for children.   3. Communicative disorders in infants. I. Title.

      [DNLM: 1. Communication Disorders—therapy—Child.   2. Communication Disorders—therapy—Infant.   3. Developmental Disabilities—therapy—Child.   4. Developmental Disabilities—therapy—Infant.   WL 340.2 R829c 2000]

      RJ496.S7 R66 2000

      618.92'855—dc21

                                        00-034508

Contents

Preface

Early interventionists representing a wide array of academic disciplines are acutely aware of the importance of targeting communication skills as an integral part of comprehensive services provided to children under the age of three. Current literature continues to support the premise that communication skills remain the single best predictor of later school success.

The first edition of this text, published in 1996, was motivated in large measure by the observation that many, if not most, early intervention (EI) professionals had not received even one class directed toward services to children under three years of age. More recent observations continue to suggest that less than 5 percent of practicing EI professionals have received sufficient coursework to prepare them to work with this unique population of children and families. These observations, as well as the wide acceptance of the first edition of this text, have prompted this second edition.

The basic premise of this edition remains the same. Specifically, communication skills must be at the center of any effective program of early intervention. Further, it does not matter who provides early intervention services; communication skills must be stressed as an integral part of the overall program of services received by children at risk for developmental pathology, or those with established risk conditions.

This edition provides updated epidemiologic information, more current efficacy data, and additional clinically relevant intervention suggestions. The content of the text is to be used by all EI professionals, regardless of primary academic discipline.

I trust that readers, regardless of primary academic discipline, will quickly note that the information presented in this second edition remains highly clinical in nature and reflects a deep respect and appreciation for all involved in the provision of early intervention services. The children and families with whom we interact deserve the best we have to offer. The purpose of this edition is to further sharpen the skills we bring to the early intervention enterprise.

Acknowledgments

I am most gratified at the need for a second edition of this text. Although the completion of the second edition was less work that the initial writing, a task of this nature necessitates the assistance of others. There are two individuals to whom I am most grateful. This past year I have had the assistance of two of the most talented graduate students I have worked with over my 26 years of university teaching. Kate Beers and Sarah Kohlenberg have worked tirelessly along side me in keeping me semi-organized and on track as this process unfolded. They are bright and hard working. Each will prove to be valuable additions to the profession once they complete their graduate studies. I wish them all the best in their careers that lie ahead.

CHAPTER

1

Populations at Risk for Communication Delay

❝ *Anything that interferes with the child's ability to interact with the environment in a normal manner is a potential source of, or contributing factor to, the presence of developmental delay.* **❞**

(Rossetti, 1990, p. 52)

Delayed communication development is the most common symptom of developmental disability in children under 3 years, affecting approximately 5% to 10% of that population. The incidence of communication delay for certain populations of infants and toddlers, specifically those with established risk factors, is substantially higher. It is generally accepted that, among all childhood behaviors, communication skills provide the highest predictive correlation with later intelligence attainment and school performance. It has been suggested that in the course of a normal day, the busy pediatrician sees at least two children under 3 years with delay in the development of communication skills (Capute & Accardo, 1978; Coplan, 1985). Hence, it is no surprise that professionals from across academic disciplines have an increased interest in the early identification of and intervention for children birth through 3 years of age who display communication delay or who are at risk of doing so.

Who are these children? What factors contribute to increased risk for communication delay and potential school difficulties? Are biological or environmental factors of primary importance when establishing risk status? Finally, are new populations of children emerging with whom the early interventionist (EI) must be concerned in order to provide comprehensive intervention services for children and their families?

These questions, although not easy to answer, are of paramount importance to the entire array of professionals interested in establishing effective intervention services for children under 3 years of age. The efficacy of early intervention, which will be discussed in greater detail in Chapter 6, depends in part on the answers to these and other questions. From a cost standpoint alone, every dollar spent on early intervention may save a school district up to $6 in later remedial services. Hence, familiarity with the population of children who display communication delay or who are at increased risk of doing so is of significant importance to the entire early intervention team.

One of the most frequently asked questions by early interventionists is, "How do I gain earlier access to children with developmental delay or those at risk of demonstrating developmental pathology?" The answer to that question is not simple. However, it is important that the EI become as familiar as possible with the wide variety of factors that contribute to developmental delay. The EI should learn to function as a broker of information regarding services for children under 3 years and their families. That is to say, the EI must be prepared to comment on many issues related to service provision for children under 3 years. Hence, the EI is encouraged to develop a database, consider who might benefit from this data, develop strategies for providing this information to decision makers relative to early intervention, and be prepared to address questions and any resistance to enhancing service provision. One principle to keep in mind is this: *Anything that interferes with a child's ability to interact with the environment in a normal manner is a potential cause of, or contributing factor to, the presence of developmental and, more specifically, communication delay.* The material following alerts all members of the early intervention team to issues that will improve the potential that all children in need of intervention and specifically communication intervention have appropriate access to services.

ESTABLISHED-RISK AND AT-RISK CHILDREN

Two concepts that the interventionist should be familiar with are established risk versus at risk for children under 3 years.

Established Risk

Children in the established-risk category have known (expected) patterns of developmental delay accompanying whatever places them in the established-risk grouping. For example, the child with Down syndrome is not considered to be at risk. This is because Down syndrome itself includes varying degrees of developmental delay affecting general intellectual functioning. Developmental delay is expected, although variation exists in long-term performance of children with Down syndrome. Variation can stem from whether a child received early intervention services, the age at which such services were received, the degree of caregiver involvement in the early intervention process, a child's general health (in particular the degree to which middle ear problems were identified and managed at an early age), and other factors.

There are a host of genetic and metabolic syndromes in which developmental delay is present. One classification system for established-risk children is employed by the state of Michigan. The Michigan system breaks established risk into nine categories, with specific conditions known to contribute to developmental delay listed under each. Following is a listing of the categories and examples of specific conditions for each. Although the listings under each category are not exhaustive, they include many of the more common established-risk factors.

Established-Risk Categories

1. Chromosomal Anomalies/Genetic Disorders

Cri-du-chat	Trisomy 21 (Down syndrome)
Trisomy 18	Fragile X syndrome
Cockayne syndrome	Laurence-Moon-Bardet-Biedl
Waardenburg syndrome	syndrome
	Cerebro-hepato-renal syndrome

2. Neurological Disorders

Cerebral palsy	Kernicterus
Progressive muscular dystrophy	Myasthenia Congenita
Paralysis	Wilson disease
Intercranial hemorrhage	Kugelberg-Welander disease
Leukodystrophies	Schildre disease
Werdnig-Hoffmann disease	Bloch-Sulzberger syndrome
Neurofibromatosis	Sturge-Weber syndrome
Intercranial tumors	Head and spinal cord injury
Seizure disorders	

3. Congenital Malformations

Patent ductus arterilsis
Transposition of great arteries
Noonan syndrome
Potter syndrome
Encephalocele
Spina bifida

Cleft palate
Hypoplastic mandible
Treacher Collins syndrome
Microcephaly

4. Inborn Errors in Metabolism

Hunter syndrome
Marqulo syndrome
Schele syndrome
Maple syrup urine disease
Galactosemia
Neimann-Pick disease
Lesch-Nyhan syndrome

Hurler-Schele syndrome
Sanfilippo syndrome
Sly syndrome
Infant PKU
Glycogen storage disease
Tay-Sachs disease
Hyper/hypo pituitary disease

5. Sensory Disorders

Visual impairment/blindness
Hearing loss

Retinopathy of prematurity
Congenital cataract

6. Atypical Developmental Disorders

Pervasive developmental
   disorder
Reactive attachment disorder

Autistic disorder
Failure to thrive (nonorganic)

7. Severe Toxic Exposure

Cocaine and other drugs
Maternal PKU

Fetal alcohol syndrome
Lead/mercury poisoning

8. Chronic Medical Illness

Medically fragile
Chronic hepatitis
Diabetes
Renal failure

Cancer
Cystic fibrosis
Heart problems

9. Severe Infectious Disease

Cytomegalovirus (CMV)
HIV positive
Syphilis
Bacterial meningitis
Poliomyelitis

Herpes
Rubella
Toxoplasmosis
Encephalitis
Viral meningitis

An excellent source of information on syndromes and metabolic disorders with established risk for developmental delay is provided by Bergsma (1979). In summary, children in an established-risk category display developmental delay secondary to the factor that places them in the established-risk category initially. Their delay is not unexpected, although many factors may be present that relate to the extent of the delay and long-term developmental expectations.

At Risk

In contrast to the child who presents established risk is the child considered to be at risk for developmental delay. An important consideration for the clinician is an understanding of the factors that contribute to the at-risk label being applied to a given infant. As was previously suggested, anything that interferes with a child's ability to interact with the environment in a normal manner is a potential cause of, or contributing factor to, developmental delay. Numerous factors interfere with normal environmental interaction and thus can increase risk for delay. These factors relate to biological as well as environmental issues. It is clear that the environment is as powerful a factor in establishing risk as biological and constitutional factors (Escalona, 1982). In many instances, the clinician is confronted with infants and toddlers at risk for displaying developmental delay from biological and environmental factors. Hence, these children are considered to be at double hazard for delay. More detailed coverage of factors that increase the risk for developmental delay is provided later in this chapter. Children at risk for substantial developmental delay are those from birth to 3 years who are at biological and/or environmental risk if early intervention services are not provided, even if signs of developmental delay are not yet observed. Once again, the state of Michigan has provided a helpful classification of risk factors. Children may be considered at risk for substantial delay based on parental and/or professional judgment and the presence of four or more of the following risk factors.

At-Risk Categories

- Serious concerns expressed by a parent, primary caregiver, or professional regarding the child's development, the parenting style, or the parent-child interaction
- Parent or primary caregiver with chronic or acute mental illness/developmental disability/mental retardation
- Parent or primary caregiver with drug or alcohol dependence
- Parent or primary caregiver with a developmental history of loss and/or abuse
- Family medical/genetic history characteristics
- Parent or primary caregiver with severe or chronic illness

- Acute family crisis
- Chronically disturbed family interaction
- Parent-child or caregiver-child separation
- Adolescent mother
- Parent with four or more preschool-age children
- The presence of one or more of the following: parental education less than 9th grade; neither parent is employed; single parent
- Physical or social isolation and/or lack of adequate social support
- Lack of stable residence, homelessness, or dangerous living conditions
- Inadequate health care or no health insurance
- Limited prenatal care
- Maternal prenatal substance abuse/use
- Severe prenatal complications
- Severe perinatal complications
- Asphyxia
- Very low birth weight (<1,500 g)
- Small for gestational age (<10th percentile)
- Excessive irritability, crying, tremulousness on the part of the infant
- Atypical or recurrent accidents on the part of the child
- Chronic otitis media

Models of Causation

The early interventionist should have an overall philosophy of causation in mind as specific factors contributing to risk are discussed. Assessment and management decisions should be made with a complete understanding of how causal factors interact and relate to a child's communication impairment. Sameroff and Chandler (1975) describe three different views of causation. These are the linear, interactional, and transactional cause-and-effect models.

Linear Cause-and-Effect Model

The linear cause-and-effect model holds that there is a direct one-to-one relationship between a cause and an effect. Inherent in this model is the necessity to determine cause because intervention and treatment arise, at least in part, from what is known about cause. This model may also be called the medical model, as this approach underlines a great deal of work in medicine. Initially this model is appealing. It prompts the clinician to search for causative factors. However, if the clinician operates under the assumption that causation determines treatment and that one cause is paramount for the pattern of delay noted in a particular child, then the model is faulty. This view is faulty because, in most instances, developmental performance, even for those children with established risk from factors previously listed, is due to a variety of circumstances. Although a child may have a specific condition known to cause developmental delay, other factors in the child's environment may likewise contribute to developmental pathology. Hence, a one-to-one view of cause and outcome is faulty.

Interactional Model

The interactional model views causation as the result of the interaction between the child's constitution and the environment. This view is more comprehensive and acknowledges the equal importance of biology and environment in contributing to developmental performance. Viewing causation in this manner indicates that a search for a single cause is unfruitful because of the interaction between biology and environment. Several limitations of the interactional model include a tendency to view biology or environmental factors as static—that is, they do not change over time. A second limitation is a failure to acknowledge that a child's environment does not affect biology and constitutional factors do not influence the environment.

Transactional Model

The transactional model of viewing causation incorporates some of the previous models but differs qualitatively from them. The transactional model includes the probability of change over time and emphasizes the reciprocal relationship between the child's environment and constitution. At the center of this model is the certainty of change over time. Thus, the child's environment may alter health status, and the child's health status may alter the environment. The application of this model is obvious. It has the clinician viewing the child's causation as being in a constant state of modification depending on the nature of the reciprocal relationship between biology and environment.

One problem with this view is that the identification of specific etiology may become more difficult. Even in the presence of clear-cut factors known to contribute to developmental delay, the exact manner in which these factors influence a child's environment is not known. Likewise, the exact manner in which environmental deficits may alter health status is not known. Thus, it is necessary for regular monitoring of the child's health and environmental status to maintain an accurate and current understanding of patterns that may be influential in the child's developmental progress or lack of progress.

One of the most frequently asked questions by clinicians desiring greater access to children under 3 years of age is, "How do I gain such access?" Enhancing service delivery to children under 3 years involves, to some degree, alerting appropriate decision makers to the need for early case finding and the effectiveness of such services. Is early intervention effective? The entire early intervention team should be able to effectively answer that question from an empirical standpoint. It is imperative that early interventionists, regardless of primary discipline, become brokers of information. That is to say, clinicians should familiarize themselves with a wide array of issues, including early case finding, populations at increased risk for communicative delay, available intervention models, efficacy, family concerns, and cost of needed services. The information following presents an epidemiologic overview of biological and environmental risk elements relating to communication impairment, plus a review of special populations of children who are emerging as at enhanced risk for developmental delay and specifically communication impairment.

Infant Mortality

Familiarity with infant-toddler mortality statistics can be of value to the clinician interested in early case finding and also when determining populations of infants and toddlers at increased risk for communication delay. Why is an understanding of infant mortality statistics important? After all, these children do not survive and consequently do not enter the interventionist's caseload. The answer to that question is relatively simple. Because of the enormous advances seen in neonatal medicine in the past decade, more infants are surviving today than ever before. Although the incidence (new occurrences per year) of low-birth-weight (LBW)/medically fragile infants has not changed dramatically in the past 5 years, the prevalence (total living cases) of medically fragile/LBW infants is expanding. As a result, the interventionist should be aware that the identical factors contributing to infant-toddler mortality also contribute to surviving infants' increased risk for developmental delay (morbidity) or match established patterns of developmental delay. In addition, expanding (new) populations of infants, such as those prenatally exposed to drugs, babies who are HIV positive, infants born to teenage mothers, and infants surviving at lower birth weights and younger gestational ages, are entering the clinician's caseload. Thus, it is important that the clinician become familiar with infant mortality, its causes and contributing factors, and various new populations of infants and toddlers to gain a full understanding of risk and long-term developmental expectations for survivors.

Each year, approximately 40,000 U.S. infants die before reaching their first birthday. Tables 1-1 to 1-3 provide an overview of births in the United States in 1997. Of all live births, 66% of infant deaths occur during the neonatal period. Of those, more than half occur to infants weighing less than 1,500 g. Infants who constitute fewer than 1% of

TABLE 1–1 Overview of Births-United States, 1997

- Every 8 seconds a baby is born in the United States.
- Every hour three babies die.
- African American infants are more than twice as likely to die before their first birthday as white infants.
- Birth defects are the leading cause of infant mortality.
- One in five infant deaths is due to birth defects.
- Every 3½ minutes a baby is born with a birth defect.
- Every 2 minutes an LBW baby is born.
- More than 3,700 babies are born weighing less than 1 pound at birth.
- Every minute a baby is born to a teen mother.
- Each day 415 babies are born to mothers who receive late or no prenatal care.
- The U.S. infant mortality rate is worse than that of 24 other nations.

Adapted from March of Dimes, 1998.

TABLE 1–2 Live Births, Infant Mortality/Rank

State	Live Births	Infant Mortality Rate	Rank
Alabama	60,329	9.8	49
Alaska	10,244	7.7	31
Arizona	72,463	7.5	27
Arkansas	35,175	8.8	40
California	552,045	6.3	11
Colorado	54,332	6.5	13
Connecticut	44,343	7.2	19
Delaware	10,266	7.5	25
D.C.	9,024	16.2	51
Florida	188,723	7.5	26
Georgia	112,282	9.4	45
Hawaii	18,595	5.8	5

(continued)

TABLE 1–2 *(continued)*

State	Live Births	Infant Mortality Rate	Rank
Idaho	18,035	6.1	8
Illinois	185,812	9.4	44
Indiana	82,835	8.4	38
Iowa	36,810	8.2	35
Kansas	37,201	7.0	18
Kentucky	52,377	7.6	28
Louisiana	65,641	9.8	48
Maine	13,896	6.5	12
Maryland	72,396	8.9	41
Massachusetts	81,648	5.2	1
Michigan	134,642	8.3	36
Minnesota	63,263	6.7	16
Mississippi	41,344	10.5	50
Missouri	73,028	7.4	23
Montana	11,142	7.0	17
Nebraska	23,243	7.4	24
Nevada	25,056	5.7	4
New Hampshire	14,665	5.5	3
New Jersey	114,821	6.6	15
New Mexico	26,920	6.2	10
New York	271,369	7.7	30
North Carolina	101,592	9.2	42
North Dakota	8,476	7.2	20
Ohio	154,061	8.7	39
Oklahoma	45,672	8.3	37
Oregon	42,811	6.1	9
Pennsylvania	151,850	7.8	32
Rhode Island	12,776	7.2	21
South Carolina	50,923	9.6	47
South Dakota	10,475	9.5	46
Tennessee	73,173	9.3	43
Texas	322,756	6.5	14
Utah	39,577	5.4	2
Vermont	6,783	6.0	7
Virginia	92,578	7.8	33
Washington	77,228	5.9	6
West Virginia	21,162	7.9	34
Wisconsin	67,479	7.3	22
Wyoming	6,261	7.7	29
Puerto Rico	63,425	12.7	
United States	3,899,589	7.6	

Adapted from March of Dimes, 1997.

TABLE 1–3   International Infant Mortality Rates (1993)

Country	Rate	Rank
Japan	4.3	1
Singapore	4.3	2
Hong Kong	4.4	3
Sweden	4.5	4
Finland	4.7	5
Switzerland	5.1	6
Norway	5.2	7
Denmark	5.5	8
Germany	5.6	9
Netherlands	5.6	10
Ireland	5.9	11
Australia	6.1	12
Northern Ireland	6.1	13
England and Wales	6.2	14
Scotland	6.2	15
Austria	6.3	16
Canada	6.3	17
France	6.5	18
Italy	6.6	19
Spain	6.7	20
New Zealand	7.2	21
Israel	7.8	22
Greece	7.9	23
Czech Republic	8.0	24
United States	8.0	25
Portugal	8.1	26
Belgium	8.2	27
Cuba	9.4	28
Slovakia	11.2	29
Puerto Rico	11.5	30
Hungary	11.6	31
Chile	12.0	32
Kuwait	12.7	33
Costa Rica	13.7	34
Poland	15.1	35
Bulgaria	16.3	36
Russian Federation	18.6	37

Adapted from March of Dimes, 1998.

Note: Includes countries that report infant mortality statistics to the World Health Organization. Rates are per 1,000 live births.

all live births account for almost 40% of all infant deaths. Major risk factors for infant mortality include the following (Hogue, Buehler, Strauss, & Smith, 1987):

- *Gender*: Regardless of race, males experience higher birth-weight-specific infant mortality than do females.
- *Gestational age*: Infant mortality decreases with increased gestational age.
- *Live birth order*: Second-born infants have lower infant mortality than infants in other birth orders.
- *Maternal age*: Infant mortality decreases with increasing maternal age through 30 to 34 years of age but increases for infants born to women 35 years of age and older. Optimal maternal age is 25 to 29 years for African American women and 30 to 34 years for white women.
- *Maternal education*: Infant mortality declines with increasing maternal education for both races but declines more steeply for infants born to white women.
- *Prenatal care*: Infants born to mothers who obtain prenatal care beginning in the first trimester have substantially lower infant mortality. This trend is most pronounced for infants weighing 2,500 g or more but is also seen in infants weighing between 1,500 and 2,499 g. Tables 1-4 to 1-8 review access to

TABLE 1–4   Percentage of Births by Entrance into Prenatal Care- United States, 1996

Trimester	Number	Percentage
First/early care	3,102,972	81.9
Second	536,401	14.2
Third/late care	106,759	2.8
No care	44,543	1.2

Total live births: 2,790,676 (excludes the 100,818 births for which prenatal care was not stated)

Adapted from March of Dimes, 1998.

TABLE 1–5   Early Prenatal Care (First Trimester)-United States, 1986-1996

Year	Percent
1986	75.9
1987	76.0
1988	75.9
1989	75.5
1990	75.8
1991	76.2
1992	77.7
1993	78.9
1994	80.2
1995	81.3
1996	81.9

Adapted from March of Dimes, 1998.

TABLE 1-6   Adequacy of Prenatal Care by Maternal Race-United States, 1996

Race	Percent Adequate Care	Percent Inadequate Care
White	74.7	10.6
African American	65.0	21.0
Native American	57.2	25.1
Asian or Pacific Islander	71.7	12.7
All races	72.9	12.4

Adapted from March of Dimes, 1999.

TABLE 1-7   Early Prenatal Care (First Trimester) by Race or Ethnic Group-United States, 1996

Race/Ethnic Group	Percentage
Total percent	82
African American	71
White	84
Puerto Rican	73
Cuban	88
Native American	67
Mexican American	63
Asian or Pacific Islander	81

Adapted from March of Dimes, 1999.

TABLE 1-8   Perinatal Statistics by Maternal Ethnicity- United States, 1996

	Mexican	Cuban	Non-Hispanic Whites	Non-Hispanic Blacks
Births	489,666	12,613	2,358,989	578,099
Births to teens	88,765	963	227,729	132,700
Low birth weight	28,691	814	149,839	75,706
Very low birth weight	7,829	170	25,365	17,419
Preterm births	50,408	1,296	222,592	100,371
Early prenatal care	337,714	11,119	2,024,891	395,966
Infant deaths	2,861	64	14,249	8,209

Note: Low birth weight <2,500 g; very low birth weight <1,500 g; early prenatal care starts in the first trimester.
Adapted from March of Dimes, 1998.

prenatal care among various groups of women in the United States.

In 1984, the U.S. infant mortality rate was 18.4 per 1,000 live-born African American infants and 9.4 per 1,000 live-born white infants. Since that time infant mortality has declined in the United States. Between 1980 and 1992, the mortality rate for white infants declined by 37% to 6.9 infant deaths per 1,000 live births, while the mortality rate for black infants declined by 24% to 16.8, widening the gap in infant mortality between the two races. However, when annual reductions in infant mortality in the United States are compared with international standards, the United States does not compare favorably. Twenty-three countries have lower infant mortality rates than the United States. The U.S. infant mortality rate is twice that of the nation with the lowest rate, Japan (Mason, 1991). The 1997 provisional infant mortality rate in the United States was 7.6 per 1,000 live births.

Diversity in U.S. infant mortality rates exists among various subpopulations (Figure 1–1). This information should be of interest to the clinician working in culturally diverse regions. From 1983 to 1985, the

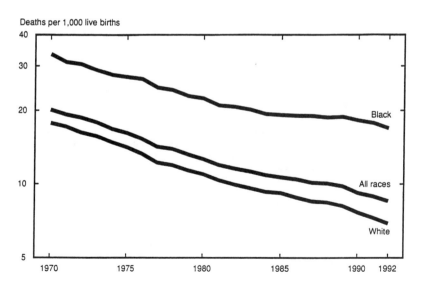

Figure 1–1   Infant mortality rates by race. (Adapted from "Infant Mortality Rates by Race," by Centers for Disease Control and Prevention, National Center for Health Statistics, 1994, *National Vital Statistics System, 23,* p. 16.)

infant mortality rate among Japanese Americans was 6 per 1,000 live births. Among Hispanics, there was wide variation in infant mortality rates. It ranged from a low of 8 among Cubans to a high of 12.3 among Puerto Ricans. Mexican Americans, the largest group, had an infant mortality rate of 8.8, which was below that of whites. The Native American rate, 13.9, and the African American rate, 18.7, were respectively 1.5 and 2.1 times the rate for whites. Figure 1–1 displays data on birth weight and gestational age for infants who are classified as appropriate versus small for gestational age. Information of this nature assists the clinician in understanding risk status for surviving infants. Table 1-9 displays 1996 data on infant mortality and maternal race.

Low Birth Weight and Prematurity

A premature infant is defined as a child born at or before the 36th week of gestation, 1 month before the ideal estimated date of delivery. A small for gestational age (SGA) infant refers to a newborn whose birth weight is below the 10th percentile for gestational age. Small for gestational age babies may have been born at term or they may have been premature. For example, a child born at 35 weeks' gestation weighing 5 lb, or 2,250 g, would be considered premature but with weight appropriate for gestational age. This weight falls at the 25th percentile for age. However, if this infant had been born at term weighing the same 5 lb he or she would be considered small for gestational age. At 40 weeks' gestational age, the 10th percentile for weight is 5½ lb, or 2,500 g.

Mortality rates are closely related to an infant's birth weight and gestational age. The most important predictor for infant survival continues to be birth weight. Hence, risk status for later developmental

TABLE 1–9   Infant Mortality by Maternal Race- United States, 1996

Race	Rate per 1,000 Live Births
White	6.1
Black	14.1
Native American	10.0
Asian or Pacific Islander	5.2
All races	7.3

Adapted from March of Dimes, 1999.

delay is likewise associated with birth weight and gestational age. Figure 1–2 displays newborn weight by gestational age and may be used in determining whether an infant is small for gestation. Tables 1-10 to 1-13 describe average fetal weight and length by gestational age as well as factors that relate to increased risk for infant mortality.

Several additional terms are helpful for clinicians gaining familiarity with infant mortality statistics. The term fetal death means death taking place at 20 weeks' gestation or later, but before birth. Perinatal death is death from 20 weeks' gestation to 27 days after birth. The neonatal time period is from birth to 27 days after birth. Infant refers to the child from birth to the end of the first year of life. Closely linked to mortality statistics is the presence or absence of an adequate level of prenatal care. Inadequate prenatal care means fewer than five prenatal medical visits for pregnancies lasting 37 weeks or longer, fewer than eight visits for pregnancies 37 weeks or longer, or

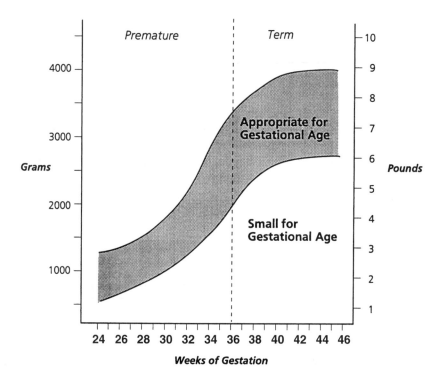

Figure 1-2   Small versus appropriate for gestational age. (Adapted from *The High-Risk Infant* (p. 59), by L. O. Lubchenco, 1976, Philadelphia: W. B. Saunders.)

TABLE 1–10   Average Fetal Weight and Size by Gestational Age

Weeks (postconception)	Weight (g)	Length (cm)
8	1	4.0
9	2	4.0
10	4	5.5
11	7	6.5
12	14	9.0
13	25	9.0
14	45	12.5
15	70	12.5
16	100	16.0
17	140	16.0
18	190	20.5
19	240	20.5
20	300	25.0
21	360	25.0
22	430	27.5
23	501	27.5
24	600	30.0
25	700	30.0
26	800	32.5
27	900	32.5
28	1001	35.0
29	1175	35.0
30	1350	37.5
31	1501	37.5
32	1675	40.0
33	1825	40.0
34	2001	42.5
35	2160	42.5
36	2340	45.0
37	2501	45.0
38	2775	47.5
39	3001	47.5
40	3250	50.0
41	3501	50.0
42	4001	52.5
43	4501	52.5

Adapted from Lubchenco, 1981.

prenatal care beginning after the first trimester of pregnancy. These concepts are of importance to the interventionist if a complete understanding of mortality and risk factors is to be gained.

TABLE 1–11   Increased Risk of
Infant Mortality

- Low and very high birth weight
- Black
- Male
- Short and long gestation
- Birth order (first and third)
- Maternal age (younger and older)
- Lower maternal education
- Lack of prenatal care

TABLE 1–12   Ten Leading Causes of Infant Mortality-
United States, 1996

Cause	Rate per 100,000 Live Births
Birth defects	164.0
Preterm/LBW	100.3
SIDS	78.4
RDS	35.0
Maternal pregnancy complications	32.1
Placenta/cord complications	24.4
Accidents	20.7
Infections	19.4
Pneumonia/influenza	12.7
Hypoxia/birth asphyxia	11.0

Adapted from March of Dimes, 1996.

TABLE 1–13   Common Medical Disorders in Newborns

- Hypoxic-ischemic encephalopathy
- Intercranial hemorrhage
- Sepsis
- Hyperbilirubinemia
- Hypoglycemia
- Inborn errors of metabolism
- Maternal substance abuse
- Seizures

Prematurity

Premature delivery is due to a number of factors, many of which are not fully understood (see Tables 1-14 and 1-15). In general, however, premature deliveries account for fewer than 5% of all live births. Fewer than 1% of these infants weigh less than 1,500 g (3.5 lb). However, this latter group accounts for 84% of all deaths in the newborn period and most of the morbidity seen in LBW infants (Avery, 1987; Klaus & Fanaroff, 1986). Although fewer than 5% of all pregnancies occur in adolescents, they account for 20% of all premature births (Goldberg & Craig, 1983). Factors that have been associated with premature delivery include poor nutrition, inadequate prenatal care, toxemia, substance abuse, and multiple births. The highest proportion of premature births is among people of lower socioeconomic groups. Thus, nonwhite underprivileged groups have nearly twice the prematurity rate as whites with higher socioeconomic status. One aspect of prematurity that should be kept in mind is the potential for recurrence. Once a mother delivers an infant prematurely, the risk of delivering another premature infant is approximately 25%. If she has delivered two premature infants, the risk of a third is approximately 70%.

TABLE 1-14   Known Causes of Prematurity

- Amniotic fluid/membrane infection
- Drug/alcohol abuse
- Fetal distress
- Maternal age (adolescent or older mother)
- Maternal chronic illness
- Maternal kidney infection/problems
- Multiple gestation
- Placental bleeding
- Poor prenatal care
- Premature rupture of membranes
- Preeclampsia
- Uterine abnormalities—incompetent cervix

TABLE 1-15   Preterm Births (Less Than 37 Weeks' Gestation)-United States, 1985-1996

Year	Percent
1985	9.8
1986	10.0
1987	10.2
1988	10.2
1989	10.6
1990	10.6
1991	10.8
1992	10.7
1993	11.0
1994	11.0
1995	11.0
1996	11.0

Adapted from March of Dimes, 1997.

Low Birth Weight

Prevention remains the best treatment option for LBW infants. In 1980 there were 3,542,995 single deliveries in the United States; in 1987 more than 3,800,000 infants were born. Between 1995 and 2000, the slowest rate of growth in United States history is projected (Spencer, 1988). Infants with birth weights of less than 1,500 g accounted for fewer than 1% of all live births but 2% of live-born African American babies. Infants in the intermediate LBW category of 1,500 to 2,499 g were 5% of all live births but 9.2% of all live-born African American births. The incidence of low birth weight (less than 2.5 kg) varies widely among different populations. In the United States, approximately 250,000 infants are born each year with weights below the 2,500 g category (Avery & First, 1989).

The past three decades have seen significant advances in neonatal medicine. This has been evidenced in improving survival rates for LBW infants. Infants between 1,500 and 2,500 g were the first group to show improved survival rates. Survival rates have been improved through transfer to intensive care nurseries, advances in respiratory support technology, enhanced methods of maintaining nutritional needs, and various drugs designed to improve survival and outcome for LBW infants. Significant changes have also been evidenced for infants below 1,500 g. More than 70% of infants below 1,500 g and 90% below 1,000 g died in the newborn period in 1960. Survivors evidenced a significant degree of developmental pathology of various forms. Only 10% were reported to be unaffected (Budetti, Barrand, & McManus, 1981). These figures have changed significantly as a result of advances in the care and treatment of LBW infants. At present, 90% of infants weighing 1,000 to 1,500 g survive. Sixty-six percent of infants in the 750 to 1,000 g range survive, and 33% of those in the 500 to 750 g range survive (Grogaard, Lindstrom, & Parker, 1990; Hack, Horbar, & Malloy, 1991). The developmental outcome of LBW and premature infants will be discussed in detail later in this chapter. Principal factors associated with risk of low birth weight are presented in Table 1-16.

Complications of Low Birth Weight and Prematurity

A variety of medical complications are generally associated with low birth weight and prematurity. That is to say, premature/LBW infants are subject to an array of complications that lengthen their hospital-

TABLE 1-16   Low Birth Weight Maternal Risk Factors

Demographic Risks
Age (less than 17, more than 34)
Race (black)
Low socioeconomic status
Unmarried
Low educational level

Risks Predating Pregnancy
Parity (0 or more than 4)
Low weight for height
Disease (diabetes/hypertension)
Nonimmune status for selected
   infections (rubella)
Poor OB history
Maternal genetic factors

Risks in Current Pregnancy
Multiple pregnancy
Poor weight gain
Short interpregnancy duration
Hypotension
Hypertension—preeclampsia—
   toxemia
First or second trimester bleeding
Placental problems
Anemia
Fetal anomalies
Incompetent cervix
Premature rupture of membranes

**Behavioral and Environmental
Risks**
Smoking
Poor nutritional status
Alcohol and other substance abuse
DES and other toxic exposures
High altitude
Inadequate or no prenatal care

Evolving Concepts of Risk
Stress: physical and psychological
Uterine irritability: events triggering
   uterine contractions
Cervical changes detected before
   onset of labor

Adapted from March of Dimes, 1997.

ization and hence contribute to the potential for later developmental pathology, including communication impairment and delay. For a detailed discussion of the physical characteristics of premature/LBW infants, see Avery (1987). A more complete discussion of the nature of the neonatal intensive care nursery and the impact of prolonged hospitalization on developmental status is contained in Chapter 2 and Chapter 4. The following information alerts clinicians to the most common complications of prematurity and low birth weight.

Respiratory Distress Syndrome

Respiratory distress syndrome (RDS) affects approximately 20% of premature infants during the first few days of life. It should be noted that respiratory problems constitute the single largest cause of death among premature/LBW infants during the neonatal period. The incidence of RDS is heavily associated with the degree of prematurity present for a particular infant. For example, 60% of infants born prior to 32 weeks' gestation are affected, compared to 10% of infants born between 34 to 36 weeks. Respiratory distress syndrome is caused by the immaturity of an infant's lungs. Depending on the level of prematurity, an infant may not possess a sufficient level of surfactant, a substance vital in preventing collapse of the lungs following each exhalation. Current treatment for RDS involves keeping the airways open, thus preventing collapse of lungs. This is accomplished by one of two methods. One method is known as continuous positive airway pressure (CPAP). In CPAP, a mixture of oxygen and air is provided under pressure through tubes placed in the nose. The second method requires intubation, which involves placing a tube down the airway and keeping the lungs inflated through the use of a ventilator. Several methods may be used following intubation to afford maximal respiratory efficiency. This method provides more direct access to the lungs and enhanced control of respiratory support. Results of these approaches in the treatment of RDS show improved survival from 50% in 1970 to 90% currently (Usher, 1987). One additional approach in the treatment of children with RDS is the use of surfactant replacement. Synthetic surfactant is now available for administration to infants with RDS. Results of surfactant administration shortly after the onset of RDS have been encouraging (Dunn, Shennan, & Zayack, 1991). The survival rate for infants treated with surfactant is approximately 65% versus 26% for children not treated (Fujiwara, Konishi, & Chida, 1990; Long, Corbet, & Cotton, 1991).

Bronchopulmonary Dysplasia

Bronchopulmonary dysplasia (BPD) is a chronic, potentially reversible lung disease of prematurely born children who have required mechanical ventilation and increased inspired oxygen concentrations in the first weeks of life. A premature infant who suffers from respiratory distress syndrome and requires oxygen for more than 28 days is generally assumed to be at substantial risk for BPD. A specific concern for infants with RDS is to provide high enough levels of oxygen, but not in excess, which increases the risk for BPD or makes it more severe. Long-term mortality after severe BPD is considerable. Sauve and Singhal (1985) report an 11.2% postdischarge mortality among infants with BPD compared to a 0.9% mortality in controls. In many infants lung function never returns to normal after BPD, and monitoring throughout life is necessary. General growth failure is common among infants with severe BPD. The reasons are probably multiple and include difficulty in providing the infants with sufficient calories, as their resting oxygen consumption averages 25% higher than comparable infants with respiratory difficulties. The increase in oxygen need is presumably from overall increased respiratory effort.

Patent Ductus Arteriosus

In approximately 30% of premature infants, normal closure of the ductus arteriosus does not take place. Gersony, Peckham, and Ellison (1983) report incidence figures between 7% for infants weighing above 1,500 g to 42% for those weighing less than 1,000 g. The ductus arteriosus connects the pulmonary artery and the aorta during fetal life. Generally, closure is stimulated by muscle contractions and oxygen intake following birth. However, in infants with respiratory difficulties, oxygen levels may not be sufficient to stimulate closure of the ductus arteriosus. These infants consequently suffer from poor ventilation as well as the open ductus arteriosus, which leads to heart failure in approximately 50% of affected infants. Two methods of treatment are available for patent ductus arteriosus (PDA). First, medication (indomethacin) may be administered. This stimulates contraction of the muscular wall of the ductus, closing it in many cases. In the event that medication is not effective in stimulating closure, a surgical procedure must be performed to close the ductus.

Apnea and Bradycardia

Apnea, a condition in which an infant ceases to breathe for periods of 20 seconds or more, and bradycardia, a deceleration in heart rate, are present in approximately 40% to 50% of infants of less than 31 weeks' gestation and in 5% to 10% of those up to 35 weeks' gestation (Avery & First, 1989). In some premature infants, apneic spells may be predictors of other patterns of disease (intercranial pathology and pneumothorax). Episodes of apnea with bradycardia (heart rate below 80 beats per minute) may result in a decrease in cerebral blood velocity with enhanced risk for additional complications. Primary treatment for apneic spells includes maintenance of lung volume, particularly in premature infants. Several drugs have been used with success (see Avery & First, 1989, p. 164). Sometimes infants respond to apneic episodes favorably with gentle rocking. A water bed may provide enough stimulus to make respirations more regular. In many instances, infants with apnea are sent home from the hospital with special monitoring equipment to assist the parents in identifying apneotic episodes. Parents are provided with instruction in cardiopulmonary resuscitation. Apnea that persists over time may be associated with more serious complications, such as brain damage. Infants who display persistent apnea and bradycardia have also been demonstrated to be at increased risk for sudden infant death syndrome (SIDS) (Batshaw & Perret, 1992).

Intercranial Hemorrhage

One of the more prominent causes of developmental pathology and neonatal mortality in LBW and premature infants is intercranial bleeding, known as intercranial/intraventricular hemorrhage (IVH). For some infants, intercranial hemorrhage is present without any obvious explanation. For others, it is associated with respiratory distress and mechanical ventilation, and with still others hemorrhages are associated with asphyxia. Intercranial hemorrhage is defined as extravascular blood within the cranial cavity (Avery & First, 1989). Intraventricular hemorrhage is an increasing problem for infants with lower birth weights who are kept alive on mechanical ventilation for respiratory distress syndrome. The general incidence of IVH is reported to be in the 35% to 45% range for infants of less than 35 weeks' gestation. The hemorrhages reach their maximum extent at about 48 hours of age. Roughly one-third of them will bleed on the first day, with the median age of onset about 16 hours. The optimum time for diagnosis by ultrasound is the end of the first week (Avery & First, 1989). In an attempt to provide a measure of severity, Papile (1979) devised a grading system for IVH. Table 1-17 presents the grades for degrees of severity of IVH. Most premature infants have some degree of IVH. When the condition is limited, outcome is generally not affected. However, if it is severe, the outcome is not good and may

TABLE 1–17   Grades for Degrees of Severity of IVH

Grade	Description
Grade I	Isolated subependymal hemorrhage
Grade II	Intraventricular hemorrhage without ventricular dilation
Grade III	Intraventricular hemorrhage with ventricular dilation
Grade IV	Intraventricular hemorrhage with parenchymal hemorrhage

Adapted from "Cerebral Intraventricular Hemorrhage (CVH) in Infants <1,500 Grams: Developmental Follow-Up at One Year," by L. Papile, 1979, *Pediatric Research, 15,* p. 528.

include mental retardation, spastic quadriplegia, and possibly hydro-cephalus. The most effective intervention for IVH is prevention. Prevention of prematurity would virtually eliminate IVH in the new-born. Other forms of treatment are described by Avery and First (1989).

Necrotizing Enterocolitis

Necrotizing enterocolitis (NEC) is a serious intestinal disorder gener-ally of preterm infants. Overall, it occurs in about 10% of infants who are less than 1,500 g at birth. Onset may occur during the first week of life. It occurs most frequently in infants with RDS and PDA. Primary treatment is discontinuation of all oral feedings. A nasogastric tube is generally utilized to prevent gastric distention. If bowel obstruction occurs, immediate surgery is needed. Mortality rates for infants with NEC range from 10% to 20%.

The information presented in the preceding section is designed to alert clinicians to the most common complications associated with low birth weight and prematurity. A variety of additional risk factors are associated with being born too soon or too small. The early inter-ventionist is encouraged to become familiar with epidemiologic issues related to mortality and morbidity for the entire population of infants that may be at risk for delay, as well as those that demonstrate established risk for developmental pathology.

New and Expanding Populations of Infants/Toddlers

Adolescent Mothers

A specific population of mothers at enhanced chance for delivering infants at increased risk for developmental delay is adolescent moth-ers. Adolescent mothers are more likely than older mothers to have LBW, premature infants, even given adequate prenatal care. This ten-dency toward low birth weight is largely because teenagers who give birth are less likely than older mothers to receive adequate prenatal care. Teenagers enrolled in good prenatal care programs can have babies with birth weights that are comparable to birth weights of babies born to mothers in their 20s. Unfortunately, in 1980, 20.1% of mothers 10 to 14 years of age and 10.3% of mothers 15 to 19 years of age received no prenatal care before the third trimester of pregnancy (Friede et al., 1987). Pregnancy among young women aged 15 through 17 showed virtually no change between 1979 and 1985, hovering around 70 per 1,000 women (Healthy People 2,000, 1990). They are also more likely to give birth to infants with disabilities. Adolescent mothers have a higher rate for spontaneous abortion, stillbirths, premature births, infants who are mentally retarded, malformations, and infants who are developmentally disabled (U.S. Department of Health and Human Services, 1980). In 1982, 13.8% of babies born to mothers under the age of 15 were of low birth weight. The percentage in 1984 was 14.5%. In 1980, there were 921,696 pregnancies among 15- to 19-year-old girls, with about 562,000 ending in live births, and 23,010 pregnancies in girls under 15 years (Centers for Disease Control, 1985; see Tables 1-18 and 1-19). As these numbers show, a strong associa-

TABLE 1-18 Common Consequences of Adolescent Childbearing

- Economic problems, lower earning potential due to higher dropout rate and child-care responsibility
- Health risks for expectant mother and child include increased incidence of STDs, toxemia, premature birth and lower birth weight, SIDS
- Social-emotional risks for mother and child
  Mother: loneliness, isolation, poor adaptation to parenting, increased incidence of child abuse
  Child: poorer adjustment to school, increased behavioral and emotional problems, poorer school performance
  Mother and child at high risk for repeating the cycle

TABLE 1–19 Percentage of Births by Maternal Age- United States, 1996

Age in Years	Percentage
40–49	1.9
35–39	10.3
30–34	23.1
25–29	27.5
20–24	24.3
18–19	7.9
15–17	4.8
<15	0.3

Total live births: 3,891,494
Total teen births: 491,577

Adapted from March of Dimes, 1997.

tion between young maternal age and increased risk of infant mortal-ity exists. Babies born to teenagers had from 1.5 to 3.5 times the risk for mortality compared with those born to mothers 25 to 29 years of age. Furthermore, African Americans had from 1.3 to 2.2 times the risk of mortality than whites, depending on maternal age (Friede et al., 1987). Figure 1–3 presents the pregnancy rate per 1,000 among adolescent girls aged 15 through 17 years. When pregnancy rates for all teenagers aged 15 to 19 years (110 per 1,000 women in 1985) are compared to rates among Hispanic women (158 per 1,000 women in 1985), Hispanic rates appear to be higher than the total population. However, Hispanic women are more likely to have married during the 15- to 19-year age range than either white or African American women.

An additional factor related to infants of teenage mothers is the type of stimulation the infant receives. Sugar (1984) reports that the percentage of adequate stimulation through mothering by adolescent

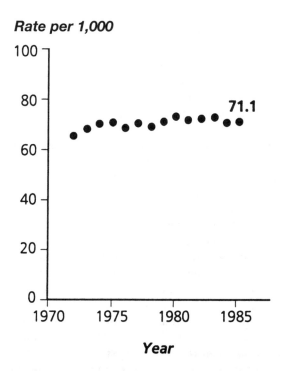

Figure 1–3   Pregnancy rate among adolescent girls ages 15 through 17. (Adapted from *Healthy People 2000*, U.S. Department of Health and Human Services, 1990, p. 73.)

versus adult mothers was 73% and 85%, respectively. For full-term infants, adequate involvement was provided by 84% of adolescent mothers versus 89% of adult mothers. It has been noted that in studying predictors of maternal involvement with premature infants (studied when the infants were 9 months of age) that education is the single best predictor. Teenage mothers, in general, have a lower overall educational level, thus suggesting that maternal involvement is somewhat lower than for adult mothers. Infants born to teenage mothers present increased risk for developmental delay (communicative delay) from a variety of biological and environmental factors. Hence, familiarity with this population of infants on the part of the interventionist is imperative.

Prenatal Drug Exposure

Approximately 5 million women of childbearing age used illegal substances in 1990. A rapidly growing body of research strongly suggests that prenatal substance exposure is linked to health problems for the newborn, as well as to problems in the child's development (Sparks, 1993). A recent study by the National Association for Perinatal Addiction Research and Education surveyed 36 hospitals in the United States and found that at least 11% of women in the hospitals studied had used illegal drugs during pregnancy (Schneider, Griffith, & Chasnoff, 1989). Based on those figures, an estimated 375,000 newborns per year face health hazards from their mothers' prenatal drug abuse.

A child exposed to drugs in utero presents with a constellation of physical, developmental, and behavioral effects, with the severity depending on the chemical substance ingested and dosage. Significant difficulty arises in monitoring the incidence of prenatal substance exposure as well as in determining the short- and long-term effects on a child's development. Perinatal problems associated with prenatal substance exposure include prematurity, stillbirth, abrupto placentae, fetal distress, intrauterine growth retardation, and low birth weight. Marijuana and cocaine are the most common illicit substances used by childbearing women. Marijuana has been associated with neonatal tremors, exaggerated startle responses, and altered visual functioning, but no characteristic physical features. Cocaine and crack, on the other hand, have been linked to potentially severe perinatal insults and central nervous system dysfunction. The physiological and behavioral consequences for the infant that survives these insults may be extreme irritability, jitteriness, tremors, seizures, hypertonia, tachycardia, tachypnea, abnormal respiratory patterns, difficulty feeding, and abnormal sleep patterns. As the infant becomes a toddler, he or she may have communication deficits, play differences, and flat emotional reactions (Russell & Free, 1991). Each of these factors contributes to increased medical and, therefore, developmental risk. Hence, determining what degree of developmental concern is from medical risk factors, what is due to exposure to various substances prenatally, and what is caused by impoverished caregiving environments becomes a formidable task. As Zuckerman (1991) has noted, the contribution of biologic variables serves to further confound follow-up on the effects of prenatal substance exposure. Factors inherent in the mother or the fetus may render some infants more vulnerable or susceptible to developmental delay. Other factors that render definitive statements regarding the effects of prenatal substance exposure difficult include the frequency and timing of the exposure. For a more complete coverage of the physical differences observed between infants prenatally substance exposed and those that were not, see Anastasiow and Harel (1993). Tables 1-20 and 1-21 further describe risks to the fetus and the baby from cocaine exposure.

In addition to the substantial risk to infants from a biological standpoint, additional risks from their caregiving environments exist. Griffith (1992) describes characteristics of cocaine-using women that have significant implications for nurturing conditions. Table 1-22 describes various characteristics of cocaine-exposed infants plus characteristics of cocaine-using women. The relationship between reduced caregiving capacity and increased needs on the part of the infant is readily apparent.

TABLE 1-20   Prenatal Exposure to Cocaine: Risks for the Fetus and the Baby

Fetal Risk	Infant Risk
Decrease in blood/oxygen flow	May display physical withdrawal
Intrauterine growth retardation	Irritability
Stroke (irreversible brain damage)	Jitteriness
Miscarriage	Disorganization
Abrupto placentae	Seizures
Neonatal neurobehavioral dysfunction	Small head circumference
Meconium staining	Premature birth
Hyperactivity	Respiratory problems
Hepatitis and HIV positive from the mother	Poor interaction ability

TABLE 1–21   Substance Abuse by Pregnancy Status of Women 15–44 Years-United States, 1994–1995

Substance	% Usage While Pregnant	% Usage Not Pregnant
Cigarettes	21.5	31.8
Alcohol	21.3	55.1
Illicit drugs	2.3	7.2

Adapted from March of Dimes, 1998.

TABLE 1–22   Characteristics of Cocaine-Exposed Infants and Mothers

Cocaine-Exposed Infants	Women Using Cocaine
Fragile	Reside in high stress environments
Disorganized	Few social supports
Low threshold for overstimulation	High degree of emotional instability
Poor regulation of states and arousal	Low self-esteem
Poor interactional capabilities	Exaggerated need for affection
	Faulty coping mechanisms
	Mothering Styles
	Detached
	Frustrated/hostile
	Overwhelmed/anxious
	Involved/overstimulating
	Involved/responsive

What is known about the long- and short-term developmental performance of drug-exposed infants and toddlers? The EI is encouraged to become familiar with these issues to enhance early case finding and improve overall service delivery to infants, toddlers, and their families. Several sources suggest that there are differences in developmental performance between drug-exposed infants and those that were not prenatally exposed to illicit substances. Free, Russell, Mills, and Hathaway (1990) report the incidence of developmental delay to be 35% for a population of drug-exposed infants that they followed over time. The greatest areas of difference are related to communication and cognitive domains. Rivers and Hedrick (1992) report differences observed in communication skills between children from birth through 6 years who were exposed to drugs and those that were not. These differences include limited expressive language, inappropriate use of gesture, reduced word retrieval ability, disorganized sentence construction, lack of turn taking, reduced pragmatic skills, limited overall vocabulary and concept formation, reduced attention span, and increased distractibility. In addition, it appears that children exposed prenatally to drugs present language delay, even in competent environments (J. Johnson, Foose, Seikel, & Madison, 1992). Full-term, cocaine-exposed infants tested at 1 month of age demonstrate depressed interactive ability and poor state control when compared to drug-free infants of the same age (Schneider et al., 1989). Four behavior patterns emerge in newborn cocaine-exposed infants. The first pattern is characterized by a lack of organization in behavioral states. The infant tends to change states rapidly from one extreme to another. The infant will enter into a deep sleep state and will not awaken in response to handling of any sort. The second pattern presents as an agitated sleep state. These infants appear stressed by external stimulation of any sort. The third pattern is characterized by vacillation between extremes of state (sleeping or crying) during handling. The final pattern is one of a panicked awake state (Schneider et al., 1989). This is reflected by a short alert period requiring caregiver help for the infant to remain calm. As these patterns demonstrate, caregiver-infant or caregiver-child interaction is considered an important foundation for the development of many later skills and is at risk in the child prenatally exposed to drugs if the caregiver is a substance abuser.

D. Johnson (1992) provides a list of basic assumptions when working with children prenatally exposed to drugs. Although not exhaustive, this list is of value to the EI in need of a philosophy about the unique challenges drug-exposed infants, toddlers, and their families pose. The basic assumptions are listed in modified form.

- Facilitating a home-school partnership is essential.
- These children are more alike than different from their peers.
- Prenatal drug exposure can cause a continuum of impairments from severe handicapping conditions to risk factors; however, there is no "typical profile."
- Behaviors seen are the outcome of a constellation of risk factors resulting from possible organic damage, early insecure attachment patterns, and ongoing environmental instability.
- Better coping skills on the part of the primary caregiver require increased self-esteem, self-control, and problem-solving ability.
- Program intervention is best achieved when all professionals concerned with the family meet on a regular schedule.

● The progress of children at risk is enhanced when they are placed in predictable, secure, and stable environments in which they can form attachments with nurturing, caring adults.

In summary, infants and toddlers prenatally exposed to drugs are at enhanced risk for neurodevelopmental delay. The exact nature of these delays has yet to be fully determined, although more information is available to the EI today than previously. Early reports, primarily in the popular media, may have significantly overstated the effect of prenatal drug exposure. Many of the behaviors noted by several researchers appear to be transient and vary from infant to infant. One area of development that appears to be deficient across populations of drug-exposed infants studied is that of communication skills. A link between play and representational (symbolic) interaction with the environment is well established. This is a population of infants and toddlers that presents deficits in symbolic interaction with the world. Hence, the potential for later communication delay and the resulting risk for school failure cannot be ignored. In addition, the caregiving environment is as equally debilitating to overall development as is prenatal exposure to illicit substances. Hence, drug-exposed infants continue to be at the higher levels of risk due to biologic and environmental factors surrounding their prenatal and caregiving circumstances.

Pediatric HIV/AIDS

In 1987 pediatric AIDS was the ninth leading cause of death in children ages 1 to 4 years and the 12th leading cause of death for children ages 5 to 14 years. As of January 1990, the Centers for Disease Control reported that 2,055 infants and children under age 13 had been reported with AIDS (Bender & Baglin, 1992). AIDS is currently one of the top five causes of death for infants and young children within the next several years (Capute & Accardo, 1996). Developmental problems for babies with HIV/AIDS appear in approximately 75% to 90% of children with HIV infection (Butler, Hittelman, & Hauger, 1991). These deficits include mental and motor delays, loss of previously acquired milestones, acquired microcephaly, short-term memory problems, cognitive deficits, fine and gross motor delays, speech and language delays, visual spatial deficits, problems with social and adaptive behavior, and attentional difficulties in older children.

The development of children with HIV infection may be confounded by other environmental and biological factors, such as prenatal drug exposure, prematurity, low birth weight, and failure to thrive. Long-term hospitalization, chaotic family environments, and understimulation may also add to the patterns of delay noted. These factors are complicated to a significant degree by the social isolation that often accompanies a diagnosis of HIV/AIDS.

To identify neurodevelopmental delays as early as possible, children with HIV infection need developmental assessment at regular intervals. One suggested pattern for assessment is provided by Butler et al. (1991). The suggested schedule for assessment includes developmental evaluation by 2 months of age, with follow-ups at least every 6 months for the first 2 years of life. After 2 years of age, children should be reevaluated at least yearly if they remain asymptomatic. If delay is identified or a decline in skills becomes apparent, more frequent evaluation may be undertaken. In older children, neurodevelopmental assessment should include tests of cognition, language, motor development, social and emotional functioning, and attention/memory skills (Brouwers, Belman, & Epstein, 1991). Once delays or deficits are recognized and fully assessed, children with HIV who are younger than 3 should be enrolled in an appropriate early intervention program. Children ages 3 through 5 should be referred to the schools for appropriate intervention services. School-age children who are HIV positive are likely to be in need of special education services (Pizzo & Wilfert, 1991). It is imperative that the EI remain current on issues related to identification and intervention for infants and toddlers with HIV/AIDS. Intervention efforts should focus on the child and the youngster's family, not the illness. The EI can serve an important role in working with pediatric HIV/AIDS in the hospital, school, and other settings of service delivery.

DEVELOPMENTAL EXPECTATIONS

Familiarity with the populations of infants and toddlers described previously in this chapter is imperative for the EI desirous of providing efficacious services. However, in addition to having an awareness of the populations listed, the EI is encouraged to become familiar with developmental expectations for the populations described. Discussion of developmental expectations becomes immediately clouded by one significant difficulty. This difficulty is reflected in the following question: Which infants/toddlers are we talking about? Although information was discussed in a more or less categorical manner, in reality, isolated categories of risk are not likely. For example, the infant born at 33 weeks' gestational age is not simply premature. That same child may be small for gestational age, experience a grade III intercranial hemorrhage, spend 76 days in the intensive care nursery, and require 30 days of assisted ventilation. Once the youngster transitions home, the caregivers may have significant difficulty in forming positive patterns of interaction and attachment and report that the child is difficult to feed and hard to comfort and has quite irregular wake/sleep patterns. Any of the categories of risk described in this chapter may apply to a particular infant. For that matter, any combination of risk factors may apply. This "continuum of risk" makes definite statements about developmental performance quite difficult. Perhaps the best manner of approaching a discussion of developmental performance is through a review of selected follow-up studies. If the EI is familiar with a broad enough sample of the populations followed, more confidence can be had in making statements about the unfolding of developmental skills.

Tables 1-23 to 1-25 are designed to provide the EI current data on developmental expectations for various populations of infants and toddlers at risk. The EI is encouraged to remain current and add to this table as new information or new populations of infants emerge. One striking fact that emerges from comprehensive study of the developmental expectations of the children discussed in this chapter is that although there is heterogeneity in the populations studied, homogeneity of outcome is present. Regardless of which population of established-risk or at-risk infants is followed, how long it is followed, which developmental domains are monitored, which assessment tools are utilized, and what biological risk factors are present, approximately 40% to 65% will display some form of developmental delay (not readily identified by standard IQ measures) into the school years.

CHAPTER SUMMARY

The first step in early case finding is knowing which infants and toddlers fall in the established-risk or at-risk category for developmental delay. The information presented in this chapter alerts the EI to factors that contribute to developmental pathology and specifically communication delay. If the most prominent feature of childhood delay is communication skill, then the EI must understand the linkage

TABLE 1-23 Developmental Expectations

Date	Authors	Population	Outcome
1987	Schraeder et al.	VLBW infants < 1,500 g	More than half of variance relative to performance at 36 months of age due to biologic factors
1989	Clark	Established-risk and at-risk babies	Problems in speech and language development observed
1990	Largo et al.	118 preterm and 78 mentally retarded infants followed to age 9 years	Language scores prior to 2 years were the strongest predictor of later performance
1986	Largo et al.	114 preterm infants followed to age 5	Language development delayed
1988	Greenberg & Crnic	30 preterm infants followed to age 2	Preterm infants significantly lower in motor skills
1985	Forslund & Bjerre	46 preterm infants followed to age 18 months	Motor, neurologic, and language development was delayed
1991	Booth et al.	18 high-risk infants followed to age 4	Attachment problems and increased aggressiveness noted
1991	Wille	18 premature, low SES infants followed to 12 months on measures of attachment	Infants were found to demonstrate insecure attachment; prematurity and low SES accounted for differences observed
1983	Wright	70 premature infants followed to age 3.5 years	Differences observed in language

(continued)

TABLE 1–23   *(continued)*

Date	Authors	Population	Outcome
			expression and comprehension compared to matched peers
1991	Blackman	Review of world's literature on LBW infants at school age	General cognitive ability within normal range; specific areas of weakness noted; underachievement, grade retention, and a need for special education more likely
1991	Hack et al.	Outcome measures on infants between 1,250 g and 1,500 g at birth	Twenty-one percent of infants followed demonstrated developmental complications
1990	Schraeder et al.	37 infants < 1,500 g followed to age 4 years	More behavior problems than would be expected in the general population
1986	Eilers et al.	43 infants < 1,250 g followed into school	More than half (51.5%) of infants followed required special education
1992	Cusson	43 high-risk, low SES infants followed to 26 months	No relationship between developmental outcome and severity of neonatal complications found
1987	Macey & Harmon	Preterm infants followed to age 12 months	Infants showed less exploratory play and stayed closer to mother during free play
1991	Oberklaid et al.	126 preterm infants followed into school	No differences observed on temperament

Date	Authors	Population	Outcome
			measures at 5 years of age
1990	Williamson et al.	61 infants < 1,500 g followed to age 1 and compared to healthy infants	Differences observed in fine motor skills; global developmental scores are not adequate in following high-risk infants
1991	Aram et al.	249 infants < 1,500 g compared with 363 normal-birth-weight infants at 8 years of age	Speech and language skills significantly lower for LBW children; language deficit and general developmental problems more prevalent
1982	Bhargava et al.	40 small for date infants compared to 40 term infants at age 1 year	Widening of gap between groups with advancing age— language differences observed between groups
1987	Hubatch et al.	10 preterm infants compared to 10 full-term infants on language skills	Superior language skills observed in full-term infants
1991	Ornstein et al.	25 studies of LBW children reviewed	Age-appropriate IQ noted; increased need for special education, visual motor problems noted, behavioral difficulties present, fine and gross motor incoordination present
1991	Escobar et al.	Review of 111 studies of LBW infants	Median incidence of disability was 25%

(continued)

TABLE 1–23　　*(continued)*

Date	Authors	Population	Outcome
1990	Grunau et al.	Infants < 1,000 g followed to age 3 years	Language outcome below that of healthy infants
1988	Vohr et al.	50 infants < 1,500 g at birth	Lower scores obtained on language tests
1993	Byrne et al.	71 LBW infants followed to age two years	Overall language scores lower than peers; 40% to 65% will display some form of developmental delay (not readily identified by standard IQ measures) into the school years

TABLE 1–24　　Birth Weight and School Performance

	Normal Birth Weight	Low Birth Weight	VLBW
Special education	3%–5%	5%–7%	13%
Repeat grade	7%	12%	25%
School failure	11%	17%	30%

Note: Normal birth weight: 2,500 g and above

Low birth weight:1,250 g–2,500 g

Very low birth weight: Under 1,250 g

between the risk factors presented and how they interact and contribute to communication delay, general developmental performance, and later school achievement. Where are the seeds for developmental delay? To some degree, enhanced potential for delay and resultant school failure begin with the presence of the factors presented in this chapter. Hence, the EI must be able to effectively communicate to decision makers that school failure does not begin when the child enters school and begins to display patterns of struggle. The seeds to school failure begin much earlier and relate in large measure to the

TABLE 1-25   Estimated Prevalence of Developmental Disorders and Other Chronic Conditions

Developmental Disorder or Chronic Disease	Cases per 1,000
Attention deficit disorder	100
Speech and language disorders	70
Learning disabilities	75
Mental retardation	20
Mild (IQ 50–70)	15
Severe (IQ <50)	5
Cerebral palsy	2
Severe hearing impairment	1.5
Autism	0.4
Visual impairment	0.4
Asthma	29
Diabetes	1
Cardiac disease	0.7

risk factors (established and at-risk) outlined in this chapter. If the EI is to truly serve as a source of information for those in decision-making positions—thereby enhancing early case finding—familiarity with the material presented in this chapter becomes imperative.

REFERENCES

Anastasiow, N., & Harel, S. (1993). *At-risk infants*. Baltimore: Paul H. Brookes.

Aram, D., Hack, M., Hawkins, S., Weissman, B., & Clark, E. (1991). Very low-birthweight children and speech and language development. *Journal of Speech and Hearing Research, 34*, 1169.

Avery, G. (1987). *Neonatology, pathophysiology, and management of the newborn* (3rd ed.). Philadelphia: J. B. Lippincott.

Avery, M., & First, L. (1989). *Pediatric medicine*. Baltimore: Williams & Wilkins.

Batshaw, M., & Perret, Y. (1992). *Children with disabilities: A medical primer* (3rd ed.). Baltimore: Paul H. Brookes.

Bender, M., & Baglin, C. (1992). *Meeting the needs of special populations*. San Diego: Singular Publishing Group, Inc.

Bergsma, D. (Ed.). (1979). *Birth defects compendium* (2nd ed.). New York: Alan Liss.

Bhargava, S., Datta, I., & Kumari, S. (1982). A longitudinal study of language development in small-for-dates children from birth to five years. *Indian Pediatrics, 19*, 123.

Blackman, J. (1991). Neonatal intensive care: Is it worth it? *Pediatric Clinics of North America, 6,* 1479.

Booth, C., Rose, K., Rubin, L., & Kenneth, H. (1991). *Journal of Social and Personal Relationships, 8,* 363.

Brouwers, P., Belman, A., & Epstein, P. (1991). Central nervous system involvement: Manifestations and evaluation. In P. Pizzo & C. Wilfert (Eds.), *Pediatric AIDS: The challenge of HIV infection in infants, children, and adolescents* (p. 82). Baltimore: Williams & Wilkins.

Budetti, P., Barrand, N., & McManus, P. (1981). *The cost and effectiveness of neonatal intensive care.* Washington, DC: Office of Technology Assessment, U.S. Government Printing Office.

Butler, C., Hittelman, J., & Hauger, S. (1991). Approach to neurodevelopmental and neurologic complications in pediatric HIV infection. *Journal of Pediatrics, 119,* 41.

Byrne, J., Ellsworth, C., Bowering, E., & Bincer, M. (1993). Language development in low birthweight infants: The first two years of life. *Journal of Developmental and Behavioral Pediatrics, 14,* 21.

Capute, A., & Accardo, P. (1996). *Development Disabilities in Infancy and Childhood.* Baltimore: Paul H. Brookes.

Capute, A., & Accardo, P. (1978). Linguistic and auditory milestones during the first two years of life. *Clinical Pediatrics, 17,* 847.

Centers for Disease Control and Prevention (1985). Teenage pregnancy and fertility trend—United States. *Journal of the American Medical Association, 253,* 3064.

Centers for Disease Control and Prevention, National Center for Health Statistics. (1994). Infant mortality rates by race. *National Vital Statistics System, 23,* 16.

Clark, D. (1989). Neonates and infants at risk for hearing and speech-language disorders. *Topics in Language Disorders, 10,* 1.

Coplan, J. (1985). Evaluation of the child with delayed speech and language. *Pediatric Annals, 14,* 203.

Cusson, R. (1992). Developmental outcome in high risk preterm infants throughout the first two years of life. *Neonatal Network, 11,* 69.

Dunn, M., Shennan, A., & Zayack, D. (1991). Bovine surfactant replacement therapy in neonates of less than 30 weeks' gestation: A randomized controlled trial of prophylaxis versus treatment. *Pediatrics, 87,* 377.

Eilers, B., Desai, N., Wilson, M., & Cunningham, D. (1986). Classroom performance and social factors of children with birth weights of 1,250 grams or less: Follow-up at 5 to 8 years of age. *Pediatrics, 77,* 203.

Escalona, S. (1982). Babies at double hazard: Early development of infants at biologic and social risk. *Pediatrics, 70,* 5.

Escobar, G., Littenberg, B., & Petitti, D. (1991). Outcome among surviving very low birthweight infants: A meta-analysis. *Archives of Disease in Children, 66,* 204.

Forslund, M., & Bjerre, I. (1985). Growth and development in preterm infants during the first 18 months. *Early Human Development, 10,* 201.

Free, T., Russell, F., Mills, B., & Hathaway, D. (1990). A descriptive study of infants and toddlers exposed prenatally to substance abuse. *Maternal and Child Nursing, 15*, 245.

Friede, A., Baldwin, W., Rhodes, P., Buehler, J., Strauss, L., Smith, J., & Hogue, C. (1987). Young maternal age and infant mortality: The role of low birthweight. *Journal of the U.S. Public Health Service, 102*, 2, 192.

Fujiwara, T., Konishi, M., & Chida, S. (1990). Surfactant replacement therapy with a single postventilatory dose of reconstituted bovine surfactant in preterm neonates with respiratory distress syndrome: Final analysis of a multicenter, double-blind, randomized trial and comparison with similar trials. The Surfactant TA Group. *Pediatrics, 86*, 753.

Gersony, W., Peckham, G., & Ellison, R. (1983). Effects of indomethacin in premature infants with patent ductus arteriosus: Results of a national collaborative study. *Journal of Pediatrics, 102*, 895.

Goldberg, G., & Craig, C. (1983). Obstetric complications in adolescent pregnancies. *South African Medical Journal, 64*, 863.

Greenberg, M., & Crnic, K. (1988). Longitudinal predictors of developmental status and social interaction in premature and full-term infants at age two. *Child Development, 59*, 554.

Griffith, D. (1992, October). *The effects of perinatal drug exposure on child development: Implications for early intervention and education.* Paper presented at the National Association for Perinatal Addiction Research and Education Conference, San Francisco.

Grogaard, J., Lindstrom, D., & Parker, R. (1990). Increased survival rate in very low birth weight infants (1,500 grams or less): No association with increased incidence of handicaps. *Journal of Pediatrics, 117*, 139.

Grunau, R., Kearney, S., & Whitfield, M. (1990). Language development at 3 years in pre-term children of birthweight below 1000g. *British Journal of Disorders of Communication, 25*, 173.

Hack, M., Horbar, J., & Malloy, M. (1991). Very low birth weight outcomes of the National Institute of Child Health and Human Development neonatal network. *Pediatrics, 87*, 587.

Healthy people 2,000: National health promotion and disease prevention objectives. (1990). *Maternal and Infant Health,* (p. 366). DHHS Publication No. (PHS) 91-50212. Washington, DC.

Hogue, C., Buehler, J., Strauss, L., & Smith, C. (1987). Overview of the National Infant Mortality Surveillance (NIMS) project—Design, methods, results. *Journal of the U.S. Public Health Service, 102*(2), 126.

Hubatch, L., Johnson, C., Kistler, D., Burns, W., & Moneka, W. (1987). Early language abilities of high risk infants. *Journal of Speech and Hearing Disorders, 50*, 195.

Johnson, D. (1992, October). *One school's experience.* Paper presented at the National Association for Perinatal Research and Education Conference, San Francisco.

Johnson, J., Foose, S., Seikel, A., & Madison, C. (1992, November). *Language abilities of 21 preschool children exhibiting cocaine intoxication at birth.* Paper presented at the Annual Convention of the American Speech-Language-Hearing Association, San Antonio, TX.

Klaus, M., & Fanaroff, A. (1986). *Care of the high risk neonate* (3rd ed.). Philadelphia: W. B. Saunders.

Largo, R., Graf, S., Kundu, S., & Hunzicker, U. (1990). Predicting developmental outcome at school-age from infant tests of normal, at-risk, and retarded infants. *Developmental Medicine and Child Neurology, 32*, 30.

Largo, R., Molinari, L., Pinto, L., & Weber, M. (1986). Language development of term and preterm children during the first five years of life. *Developmental Medicine and Child Neurology, 28*, 333.

Long, W., Corbet, A., & Cotton, R. (1991). A controlled trial of synthetic surfactant in infants weighing 1250 grams or more with respiratory distress syndrome. *New England Journal of Medicine, 325*, 1696.

Lubehenco, L. (1981). *Gestational age, birth weight and the high risk infant.* Johnson & Johnson Baby Products, Baltimore, MD.

Lubehenco, L. (1976). *The high risk infant.* Philadelphia: W. B. Saunders.

Macey, T., & Harmon, R. (1987). Impact of premature birth on the development of the infant in the family. *Journal of Consulting and Clinical Psychology, 55*, 846.

Mason, J. (1991). Reducing infant mortality in the United States through "Healthy Start." *Public Health Reports, 106*(5), 479.

Oberklaid, F., Sewell, J., Sanson, A., & Prior, M. (1991). Temperament and behavior of preterm infants: A six year follow-up. *Pediatrics, 87*, 854.

Ornstein, M., Ohlsson, A., Edmonds, J., & Asztalos, E. (1991). Neonatal follow-up of very low birthweight/extremely low birthweight infants to school age: A critical overview. *Acta Pediatrica Scandinavia, 80*, 741.

Papile, L. (1979). Cerebral intraventricular hemorrhage (CVH) in infants <1,500 grams: Developmental follow-up at one year. *Pediatric Research, 15*, 528.

Pizzo, P. (1990). Pediatric AIDS: Problems within problems. *Journal of Infectious Diseases, 161*, 316.

Pizzo, P., & Wilfert, C. (Eds.). (1991). *Pediatric AIDS: The challenge of HIV infections in infants, children, and adolescents* (1st ed.). Baltimore: Williams and Wilkins.

Rivers, K., & Hedrick, D. (1992). Language and behavioral concerns for drug-exposed infants and toddlers. *Infant-Toddler Intervention, 2*, 63.

Russell, F., & Free, T. (1991). Early intervention for infants and toddlers with prenatal drug exposure. *Infants and Young Children, 3*, 78.

Sameroff, A., & Chandler, M. (1975). Reproductive risk and the continuum of caretaking casualty. In F. Horowitz (Ed.), *Review of child development research: Volume 4* (p. 97). Chicago: University of Chicago Press.

Sauve, R., & Singhal, N. (1985). Long-term morbidity of infants with bronchopulmonary dysplasia. *Pediatrics, 76*, 725.

Schneider, J., Griffith, D., & Chasnoff, I. (1989). Infants exposed to cocaine in utero: Implications for development assessment and intervention. *Infants and Young Children, 1*, 25.

Schraeder, B., Herverly, M., & Rappaport, J. (1990). Temperament, behavior problems, and learning skills in very low birth weight preschoolers. *Research in Nursing and Health, 13,* 27.

Schraeder, B., Rappaport, J., & Courtwright, L. (1987). Preschool development of very low birthweight infants. *Journal of Nursing Scholarship, 19,* 174.

Sparks, S. (1993). *Children of prenatal substance abuse.* San Diego: Singular Publishing Group, Inc.

Spencer, G. (1988). Projections of the population of the United States, by age, sex, and race: 1988 to 2080. *Current Population Reports, Population Estimates and Projections.* Series P-25, No. 1018. Washington, DC.

Sugar, M. (Ed.). (1984). *Adolescent parenthood.* New York: S. P. Medical & Scientific Books.

U.S. Department of Health and Human Services. (1980). *Report to the president. Prevention strategies that work.* President's Commission on Mental Retardation. Washington, DC: U.S. Government Printing Office.

Usher, R. (1987). Extreme prematurity. In G. Avery (Ed.), *Neonatology* (3rd ed.) (p. 113). Philadelphia: J. B. Lippincott.

Vohr, B., Garcia-Coll, C., & Oh, W. (1988). Language development of low birthweight infants at 2 years. *Developmental Medicine and Child Neurology, 30,* 608.

Wille, D. (1991). Relation of preterm birth with quality of infant-mother attachment at one year. *Infant Behavior and Development, 14,* 227.

Williamson, D., Wilson, G., Ligschitz, M., & Thurber, S. (1990). Nonhandicapped very-low-birth-weight infants at one year of age: Developmental profile. *Pediatrics, 30,* 405.

Wright, N. (1983). The speech and language development of low birth weight infants. *British Journal of Disorders of Communication, 18,* 187.

Zuckerman, B. (1991). Drug-exposed infants: Understanding the medical risk. *The Future of Children, 1,* 26.

CHAPTER

2

Enhancing Caregiver-Infant Attachment, Interaction, and Socio-Communicative Development

❝ Attachment is a unique relationship between two people that lasts over time. For proper attachment to form, two things are necessary. These are opportunity and ability. Any interference in these, for the infant or the caregiver, may contribute to deficits in interaction patterns and communicative performance. ❞

Children do not learn to communicate in a laboratory, but rather through naturalistic interactions with their environment. The process begins early and requires a healthy start, sufficient opportunity, and exposure to a caregiving environment that allows the child's innate predisposition to learn to communicate ample opportunity to function. The children described in the previous chapter do not have a healthy start and, as a result, are not afforded early optimal opportunity to interact with their world. Hence, increased potential for developmental delay is present for such children.

Although significant attention has been directed toward infants, particularly in light of improving survival, less attention has been placed on caregivers and the impact of having an ill child with an array of medical risk factors associated with illness. In other words, only recently has attention been directed toward the caregivers of the at-risk infants and infants with disabilities described in the previous chapter.

How are their lives changed, and what adjustment difficulties do they face? Do these difficulties translate into caregiving struggles, and is an increased risk of communication deficit present if early attachment/interaction is not optimal? These are issues that the EI must address if caregivers are to be full partners in the early intervention process. Anything the EI can do to increase caregiver involvement in intervention will benefit the child and improve long-term developmental expectations. The information in this chapter alerts the EI to the unique difficulties faced by caregivers of infants and toddlers with special needs. Suggestions about how the children's adjustment may be facilitated are provided and examples given.

Regardless of primary academic discipline, all members of the EI team should be familiar with the range of challenges that face caregivers following the birth of a premature or medically fragile child. This familiarity readily translates into clinically relevant and helpful intervention suggestions for caregivers, who face the significant hurdle of developing optimal patterns of attachment and interaction once the child is in the home setting. The result is better communication skills and an overall developmental outcome more favorable than if these patterns of attachment and interaction are not fully developed.

CASE STUDIES

Perhaps the most effective manner in which the EI can gain a more complete understanding of the issues faced by caregivers of sick and at-risk infants and how these issues relate to attachment and interaction is to review the following case studies. The information in these case studies is not unique. The situations described are representative of many similar cases for which the author has provided intervention services.

The Twins

In April 1992 Mark and Jan gave birth to twin sons, Philip and Peter. The boys were delivered 9 weeks early, weighing 1,100 and 1,020 g, respectively. The boys were delivered in a regional prenatal center and were immediately placed in the neonatal intensive care nursery (NICU). Mark is a salesman and Jan is a homemaker. Mark is from the midwestern United States and Jan is from Laos. They met in Laos while Mark was on a short-term assignment. Jan's English skills are limited. Both boys were placed on assisted ventilation and appeared to be relatively healthy given their degree of prematurity and low birth weight. On day 4, Peter's condition deteriorated and it was determined that he was in need of the services of a pediatric cardiologist. As a result, he was transferred to a major university-related teaching hospital 90 miles from his home. Mark and Jan's daily routine quickly became emotionally and physically exhausting.

Jan spent the bulk of her day in the local NICU with Philip. Mark, after finishing work at 4 P.M., drove 2 hours to spend as much time as possible with Peter. He remained with Peter until midnight and drove home, arriving at approximately 2 A.M., returning to work the next day. This was Mark's routine 5 days per week. Jan saw Peter infrequently during his time away from her. She displayed a significant amount of fear, guilt, and anxiety about the boys' condition and future. Slowly, Philip's condition improved, while Peter's worsened. Jan, although afforded maximal opportunity to provide care for Philip while he was in the NICU, declined to do so. She indicated that she was fearful, and being a first-time mother, was quite overwhelmed by the nature of the NICU. As Peter's condition worsened, Jan spent less and less time with Philip, choosing instead to stay home. Mark continued his daily routine of visiting Peter and attempted to spend whatever time he could with Philip.

On day 26, Peter died. On day 38, Philip was dismissed from the NICU. The transition home for Mark and Jan was difficult, especially for Jan. She continued to struggle with guilt and fearfulness relative to her caregiving ability. Both Mark and Jan were provided with caregiver-related services when the boys were hospitalized. Mental health professionals were made available to them. After Philip transferred home, early intervention services were initiated. Two weeks after Philip's release from the hospital, the author received a phone call from Jan. The call came at 11 P.M. on a Sunday evening. She asked a very simple question, one that in large measure exemplifies the unique set of circumstances caregivers such as Jan and Mark face. Her question was simple, yet profoundly powerful. She asked, "Can you help me? I am having trouble loving my baby."

The Dad

Bill was a PhD-level family therapist who worked in a local mental health facility. He and his wife, Paula, had three sons. The boy's ages were 26, 24, and 21 years. Bill grew up on a farm in the Midwest and recalled with fondness the endless hours he spent with his father

involved in farming chores. Many years previously, as he had anticipated marriage and raising a family of his own, he determined that he
would expend whatever energy necessary to build the same degree of
closeness with his children that he had experienced with his father. To a
large extent, he felt that he had accomplished this with two of his sons.

The birth of their third son, Scott, presented Bill and Paula with
an unexpected set of trials. Scott was born at approximately 32 weeks'
gestation, weighing 1,350 g. This was considered relatively small at
the time of his birth (21 years ago). Bill and Paula were informed that
Scott had approximately a 50% chance for survival. The hospital routine followed at that time did not afford them the amount of time they
desired with Scott.

To everyone's surprise, including the physicians, Scott demonstrated slow but steady improvement. He was dismissed from the hospital on day 37. Bill and Paula felt they were taking home a "stranger."
At this point, 21 years later, Bill recalls the difficulty he had in developing the type of relationship with Scott that he had with his other sons.
He indicated that although he and Scott are close, there remains something "qualitatively different" about the nature of the relationship. Bill
attributes this "difference" to the lack of opportunity he had with Scott
during the weeks following his birth, as well as anxiety about their parenting ability in light of Scott's fragile early weeks of life. Bill's evaluation of his feelings is that even relatively short-term interruptions in
caregiver opportunity to provide ongoing early care for a child may
translate into long-term variations in the type of relationship that
develops between children and their caregivers.

The Adolescent Mother

As was noted in the previous chapter, children born to teenage mothers face a unique set of medical and caregiving risks. This set of risks
is enhanced in the presence of additional complications, such as those
displayed by Sarah.

Sarah is a 15-year-old African American mother. She has a history
of inadequate prenatal care and admits to frequent drug usage during
her pregnancy. Her daughter, Latisha, was born cocaine addicted at
approximately 30 weeks' gestation, weighing 1,020 g. The author met
Sarah during a consultation provided in a large teaching hospital.
Latisha was 26 days of age on the day of the consultation. Sarah's
mother (the baby's grandmother) was present and indicated that she
wanted nothing to do with Latisha. The mother's response was, "She
went and had a baby, now she has to take care of it. I don't want to be

bothered by it." Sarah was completely overwhelmed by the nature of the NICU. Her fear was displayed by a stony silence that prevented all but the most basic communication with her.

Prior to day 26, Sarah had been put in contact with early intervention personnel in the NICU. A program of parent training was begun, and Sarah was encouraged, even required, to provide an increasing amount of care for her daughter while in the NICU. The nursing staff indicated that Sarah was demonstrating an increasing "investment" in the child's care. Although this investment was not as consistent as they would have liked, it was present.

During the consultation it was learned that Latisha's medical condition was steadily improving. Although an exact date of dismissal could not be determined, discharge planning, from a medical and early intervention standpoint, had already begun. Sarah was asked what her greatest fear was as she anticipated taking Latisha home. She indicated that she was most concerned about two things. First, she was fearful about Latisha's medical condition and whether her use of drugs was going to harm Latisha for the rest of the child's life. And second, she was fearful that she would not be able to remain free from drug usage herself.

At this time, it is not known whether Sarah has returned to school or has received needed drug rehabilitation services. Latisha's developmental and health status is also unknown.

Summary

Each of the case studies presented above illustrates different challenges for the early interventionist. Each case points out the unique set of circumstances that caregivers face when their child is born early, ill, or at environmental risk for ongoing developmental delay. The following material is designed to provide the EI with a broad discussion of issues surrounding the difficulties inherent in forming appropriate attachment and interaction for at-risk infants and infants with disabilities and how these issues relate to caregiver participation in intervention services.

FOUNDATIONS OF NORMAL ATTACHMENT

The infant-mother attachment relationship has become the focus of a growing proportion of child development research during the past decade. This is particularly true for those infants born ill, early, or at increased risk for attachment disorders. What emerges is a consistent description of the importance of early opportunity for proper attachment to develop. That intimate contact between a woman and her newly born child influences her later behavior toward the child has been well accepted by researchers representing various disciplines (Ali & Lowry, 1981; Crawford, 1982; Goldberg, 1990; Goldson, 1992; Provence, 1990; Ross, 1980; Taylor & Hall, 1979). This section is designed to provide the EI with a basic understanding of the process of attachment, the relationship between attachment and interaction patterns between infant and mother, and barriers to proper attachment, and it gives suggestions for intervention geared toward improving attachment, interaction, and later communicative performance.

Prenatal Attachment

The process of attachment can be described as taking place both prior to and following birth. Klaus and Fanaroff (1979) describe a nine-step process in the formation of proper attachment. These steps are planning the pregnancy, confirming the pregnancy, accepting the pregnancy, fetal movement, accepting the fetus as an individual, birth, seeing and hearing the baby, touching and holding the baby, and caretaking. Although there may be variations from mother to mother, five of the nine steps described take place before birth.

Many women initially report negative or ambivalent feelings about their pregnancy. The experience of "quickening" (fetal movement) appears to be important during prenatal attachment. Although mothers may not recall the exact date or place they experienced "quickening," they can recall general details of the first instance of fetal movement. A range of thoughts enters the mother's mind during this part of the pregnancy. These thoughts include ongoing fantasies about the child to be, fears for the infant's and her own health, and the long-term changes that the birth of the child will bring to her life. Although most women report various fears regarding their child's health, few women report that they became engulfed in fear and could not place it in proper perspective. The mother begins to recognize the growing fetus as a separate individual. The mother transitions from viewing the fetus as part of her to a separate individual that will one day possess very individual characteristics apart from herself.

As suggested earlier, the experience of fetal movement is important in that it represents the child's first contribution to the parent-child relationship. From the middle of the pregnancy on, a mother becomes increasingly familiar with her child's cycles and rhythms. The child likewise becomes familiar with the mother's wake/sleep cycles and shows evidence of modifying its behavior level to maternal activity patterns. Thus, another component of synchrony between infant and mother is initiated.

Although there is not a great deal of information on a timetable for attachment, McFarlane (1978) reported that 41% of British women became attached (felt that their baby was theirs) prior to delivery. Hence, the importance of the gestational period to attachment and preparing the mother for the impending birth of her child is well established.

Parents lose much when their infant is born early, ill, or presenting any of the medical factors described in the previous chapter. The preparatory work completed during the last trimester of pregnancy is abruptly interrupted with a premature delivery. A complete opportunity for the mother to develop prenatal attachment is not possible in many instances. Much discussion has been directed toward the effect on the baby of being born before term. In a discussion of attachment, it must be recalled by the EI that much is lost to the mother as well.

Postnatal Attachment

As was previously noted by McFarlane (1978), more than 50% of mothers indicate that they became attached to their infant following birth. Clearly, the importance of the early minutes following birth plus the following days and weeks, relative to the formation of optimal attachment, is well established. In instances in which the mother is not allowed early contact with her infant, a loss of optimal attachment may result. Evidence of a sensitive period for the mother relative to the formation of proper attachment is available from a variety of sources (Klaus & Kennell, 1976; Klaus, Leger, & Trause, 1982; Rossetti, 1990). Thus, early opportunity for the mother and baby to get to know one another is essential for the process of attachment to begin.

Two significant factors following the birth of an infant should be stressed. These relate to issues of postnatal attachment. First, during the first 60 to 90 minutes after birth, the healthy infant is alert, responsive, and especially appealing. In fact, the child may be more alert during the first 60 to 90 minutes following birth than during the next 6 to 8 hours. Second, it is interesting to note that women from around the world, regardless of age or birthing practices, tend to have the same response following the birth of their child. Most women ask about the sex and health status of the child immediately following the child's birth. Following this, women request to see the child. Comments such as "Let me see my baby; Come see me; Let me look at you; Come see mother; Let me see your eyes; Come to me" are very common. It would appear that the infant and the mother are displaying behaviors following birth that set into motion the process of postnatal attachment. For the process to continue, ample opportunity and ability for the mother and the infant must be present. Two phases in the process of attachment are worth mentioning at this point. These are seeing-touching, holding the baby, and caretaking.

Seeing, Touching, and Holding the Baby

In most instances, hearing and seeing the baby begins immediately after birth. Initial interest in making visual contact with the baby causes parents to align their face in the same parallel plane as their infant. Eye-to-eye contact between mother and infant results in the initiation of maternal caretaking responses. The cry of the infant likewise affects maternal responses. A high percentage of mothers demonstrate increased blood flow to their breasts on hearing the hunger cries of their newborns. Soon after birth, if given sufficient opportunity, mothers demonstrate an ability to identify their baby's cry from others. Mothers will demonstrate a significant drive to attract their baby's attention and keep it for as long as possible following birth. It is apparent that there is a predictable pattern of responses demonstrated by a mother following birth that set in motion the early stages of attachment formation. For the process to begin, the mother must be allowed to see and initially interact with her baby. In addition, the baby must respond to her in a manner that reinforces the effort she puts forth to get to know her child.

Following initial visual contact with the baby, touching and holding become critically important in the initial stages of attachment formation. Initial touching of the infant by the mother involves use of the fingertips in stroking the infant's extremities. The touch progresses to massage and stroking of the child's trunk with the palm of the hand. Similar behavior has been noted in fathers as well. The importance of early touch is evidenced by the change in birthing procedures that have taken place in the United States during the past 25 years. Most hospitals now allow the mother maximal opportunity to interact with her newborn following birth. Many hospitals allow "rooming in." This gives the mother the opportunity to provide all or most of the needed care the infant requires before discharge home. An increasing number of women are returning home on the same day that the child is born. This also allows the mother maximal freedom in providing early care for her child. Regardless of the setting in which the child is born, a consistent picture of maternal and infant response patterns is evident.

Caretaking

Early caretaking provided by the mother is perhaps the most important factor in the formation of optimal attachment. It is through the normal daily routines of caring for a newborn that the mother fully invests herself in the child's care. In addition, regular contact of this nature allows the mother to learn the child's rhythms, distress signals, and interaction patterns. There is no substitute for early caretaking in affording the mother an opportunity to get to know her baby and for the baby to identify and respond to its mother.

During the process of caretaking, the child makes a variety of demands on the caretakers. The degree to which these demands are met has long-lasting implications for later attachment and interaction patterns. Caretaking involves three basic steps. First, the infant makes a demand. The demand may be expressed in several forms (usually crying or fussing) and may represent one of several needs. These needs may include hunger, loneliness, discomfort, fear, and the need for a change in position or location. Second, the parent attempts to meet the child's demands. It is imperative that the caretakers have opportunity to experience the manner in which their baby makes demands, how to best meet the child's needs, and how to interpret the signals the child sends them. Parents of premature and hospitalized infants who do not have early caretaking opportunity regularly report that they feel they are taking a "stranger" home when the child is dismissed from the hospital. Finally, the infant responds to the caretaker's attempts to meet expressed demands. The response may be one of pleasure and contentment or of continued discomfort. It is at this time that the caretaker may experience frustration due to the inability to meet the child's demands. If the parent receives a negative response to caretaking attempts, increased anxiety may develop. If the parent receives a positive response to caretaking activity, a strengthening of attachment may result, and caregiver confidence is increased.

For healthy infants and involved caregivers, attachment is the natural result of caretaking opportunity. However, there can be many barriers to the formation of proper attachment. These barriers and suggestions for intervention are discussed later in this chapter.

MATERNAL-INFANT INTERACTION AND COMMUNICATIVE DEVELOPMENT

Information presented in the previous chapter identified communication as the developmental domain most likely to be deficient for infants and toddlers who are at risk and/or disabled. Why is the development of communication at such enhanced risk for these children? It must be recalled that environmental and biological factors contribute to patterns of communication delay. However, the impact of deficient attachment and interaction patterns cannot be underestimated. Lack of opportunity for early contact between mother and infant, the medical condition of the child, caregiver adjustment difficulties, and various other factors play a role in the formation of less-than-optimal interaction patterns between infant and mother.

Brazelton and Cramer (1990) outline six characteristics of parent-infant interaction. Although additional paradigms exist for the delineation of interaction, the Brazelton and Cramer description lends itself readily to intervention suggestions for parents displaying deficient interaction patterns. Each of these characteristics is briefly discussed.

1. *Synchrony*: This stage involves the parents' adapting their behavior to the rhythms of the child. As the child's needs are met, caregiver confidence is increased and the parents learn to read the child's cues.
2. *Symmetry*: This second stage includes parental respect (identification) for the child's threshold for stimulation in a given interaction. The parent must recognize the child's capacity for attention, interaction styles, and preferences for interaction.
3. *Contingency*: At this point, the parents are more fully aware that their desire to interact with the child depends in large measure on the child's desire to mutually interact. The child's overall state and needs in part dictate parental success in interaction.
4. *Entrainment*: This step is accomplished once the infant and parent establish a rhythm of interaction. This is fully accomplished when the infant and parent understand each other's styles of interaction.
5. *Play*: Play is important in that it marks a period when the child learns that he or she can have increasing control over caregivers, based on the youngster's response patterns. The caregiver generally

introduces pleasurable, repetitive patterns of interaction, which expand as interaction styles evolve.

6. *Autonomy*: This step is accomplished over time as the child becomes more aware of the control he or she has over interactions that take place between the child and the caregiver.

The importance of the process described by Brazelton and Cramer (1990) relative to the development of communication skills cannot be understated. The EI should be familiar with the potential that interruptions in this process, present for many at-risk infants, may have short-term and long-term implications for the development of communication skills.

Interaction

Longitudinal study has pointed to the power of the postnatal environment in influencing the development of at-risk infants and toddlers. This is particularly true in the area of communication development. What emerges from investigations designed to monitor interaction patterns between mothers, fathers, and at-risk infants is a consistent pattern differentiating between healthy and ill infants and their parents/caregivers. The ongoing process of social interaction between caregiver and infant has the potential of minimizing or maximizing the effects of any prenatal or postnatal difficulties. Optimal child development is a process that is characterized by the interaction of biological and environmental factors. Hence, human relationships are crucially important for a child's physical, cognitive, and emotional development and for his or her full participation in society and culture (Provence, 1990). Varied forms of expression of comfort, discomfort, pleasure, and protest are generally recognizable from early infancy. Although these responses are based on biological necessity, they are subject to social learning, beginning with the earliest reciprocal interchanges between caregiver and infant. Thus, what goes on between a child and those closest to the infant is a critical influence on development, in general, and in specific developmental domains (communication). Infants and caregivers who are able to form optimal patterns of interaction (synchrony) increase potential for appropriate communication development (Sparks, Oas, & Erickson, 1988). Mothers and infants, through mutual exchange (interaction), respond to each other on a variety of social and sensory levels. To a significant degree, this exchange forms the basis upon which later communication development depends. Infants come into the world uniquely pre-disposed to interact with it. In most instances, this predisposition is coordinated with the caregivers' readiness to meet the child's needs and begin the process of attachment and interaction. The child at risk, from biologic and/or environmental factors, interacts with the world differently. Likewise, the parent of the at-risk infant interacts with the child differently. These factors contribute to the patterns of communi-cation delay noted for a high percentage of at-risk infants.

Infant Patterns of Interaction

Close study of interaction patterns among various populations of at-risk infants reveals differences when compared with patterns for healthy, full-term infants. The ill infant, premature or otherwise, is immature and demonstrates a less organized orientation to the envi-ronment. This is characterized by immature motor patterns, excessive tuning out of stressful stimuli, and lessened ability to self-regulate state (Goldson, 1992). These differences may persist into the first year and beyond. Als and Brazelton (1981) followed a group of 10 prema-ture infants for a 9-month period. Their overall findings demon-strated that the premature infants were far less responsive and much more disorganized in all of their interactions than were full-term infants. Longer-term follow-up (Bakeman & Brown, 1977) revealed similar findings. At 3 years of age, the followed population of prema-ture infants demonstrated continued inferiority in social peer interac-tions. Additional studies have pointed to the premature infants' decreased awake time, difficulty in processing environmental stimuli, generally disorganized behavior, and temperamental differences (Brown & Bakeman, 1980; Field, 1977; Field, 1980a; Rose, 1983). Table 2–1 presents information relative to a 14-month follow-up study of premature infants' interaction styles (Crawford, 1982). What is seen is a consistent pattern differentiating preterm from full-term infants on several behaviors used to monitor interactions. It should be noted that the results of the Crawford investigation revealed that preterm infants demonstrated performance closer to that of full-term infants as the children increased in age. However, premature infants did not vocalize as frequently as full-term infants throughout the 14 months of follow-up. This finding is significant in looking at the development of communicative skills for at-risk infants.

Supporting data is supplied by Field (1983). Table 2–2 presents differences in interaction behaviors between preterm and term

TABLE 2-1 Group Differences in Behavior by Chronological Age (Frequency in %)

Behavior	Age in Months							
	6		8		10		14	
	FT	PT	FT	PT	FT	PT	FT	PT
Vocalizes	15.8	23.5*	22.3	27.2*	23.0	28.6*	25.7	33.5*
Looks at objects	35.2	25.3*	36.7	22.7*	33.4	20.9*	28.4	22.5*
Looks around	16.0	12.9*	17.4	11.9*	13.5	8.1*	2.2	1.7*
Frets/cries	16.6	8.7*	11.0	8.8*	12.6	7.2*	6.4	8.1*
Plays with objects	17.5	43.8*	37.0	57.3*	50.1	73.0*	68.9	74.8*

Note: FT denotes full-term infant; PT denotes preterm infant.

* Denotes statistically significant difference

Adapted from "Maternal-Infant Interaction in Premature and Full-Term Infants," by J. Crawford, 1982, *Child Development, 53,* p. 957.

TABLE 2-2 Mean Frequency of Behaviors: Term Normal Compared to Preterm Infants (Frequency in %)

Infant Behavior	Term/Normal	Preterm
Happy	7.8	2.0
Sad	0.4	4.1
Interested	5.8	4.3
Vocalization	4.9	2.4
Crying	0.0	3.0
Expressivity rating	3.3	1.5

Adapted from "High Risk Infants Have Less Fun during Early Interactions," by T. Field, 1983, *Topics in Early Childhood Special Education*, 3, p. 77.

infants. The term infants exhibited significantly more happy faces than did the preterm infants. The preterm infants showed sad faces more frequently. Supportive caregiver responses to pleasurable infant reactions are more likely to take place and increase over time. Conversely, negative infant reactions are likely to result in less vigorous attempts on the caregiver's part to engage the infant in pleasurable interactions. Data on infant vocalizations suggested that cooing occurred more frequently among normal infants and that crying was observed more among the preterm infants. Contingent smiling occurred more frequently among healthy infants than among the preterm infants. Overall, on measures of expressivity, the group of term infants received more positive expressivity ratings than did the preterm infants. The overall results of this investigation indicated that the high-risk infants have less fun during early interactions. They were less attentive to their mothers and smiled and vocalized less frequently. These findings suggest a relationship between the patterns of delayed communication seen in high-risk infants and early infant interaction patterns.

Infants and toddlers who are at risk and disabled interact with their world and their caregivers in a quantitatively and qualitatively different fashion than do healthy children. These patterns depend, at least in part, on the biological factors for each infant. Early experience available to an infant plays a significant role in overall development. If biological factors restrict a child's exposure to its world or the ability to interact with it, there are short- and long-term implications for the development of age-appropriate communication skills.

Caregiver Patterns of Interaction

A mother's interaction with her infant is in part influenced by the infant's contribution to their relationship. Infants help their caregivers feel and be effective by being readable, predictable, and responsive. What has been noted thus far is that ill infants interact with their world in a different fashion than do healthy infants. These differences, although initially related to biologic factors surrounding an illness, frequently translate into learned behaviors reinforced by the caregivers' responses. This becomes an area of significant interest for the EI. How do caregivers and parents interact with their sick children? Can intervention be provided that improves interaction patterns and thereby enhances communication development? Although ill infants evoke caregiving responses from their mothers, the responses differ quantitatively and qualitatively from those elicited by healthy children. The nature of these differences is explored in the following information.

Altered behavioral responses in ill infants have an effect on the interaction patterns displayed by their mothers. This is important in that researchers have linked dissimilar interaction styles with later differences in cognitive behavior. Even short-term interruptions in caretaking opportunity increase the potential for impaired caretaker interactions with an infant. Ross (1980) has suggested that early contact during the first 1 or 2 hours after delivery results in more affectionate behaviors such as face-to-face looking, kissing, and fondling until at least 1 year of age. Mothers of ill infants demonstrate interaction patterns characterized by increased anxiety, stress, and depression (Oehler, Hannan, & Catlett, 1993). Mothers of ill infants consistently report that they cry more, feel guilty, and worry more than do mothers of healthy children. Even following an ill child's discharge from the hospital, caregivers report emotional upset, disappointment in the child's appearance, a sense of alienation, and concern about survival and later development (Pederson, 1987). These factors certainly have the potential to influence maternal interaction with a child.

Studies of early interaction patterns between mothers and infants found that mothers of ill infants used and sought the face-to-face position less and smiled less with their infants (Minde, 1983). Follow-up studies conducted when the child reached several months of age show that mothers were less responsive to infant cues, tended to be overactive, demonstrated less affective behavior, talked less frequently to the child, and showed less affection (Minde, Perotta, & Martin, 1985; Field, 1977; Zarling, Hirsch, & Landry, 1988).

Although specific aspects of interaction behaviors differ from mother to mother, early events certainly appear to influence maternal involvement in establishing a mutually pleasurable style of interaction. In optimal circumstances, infant responses elicit caretaking behaviors by the mother that set in motion the process of attachment and interaction. The presence of illness, lack of opportunity to care for the child, ongoing illness, maternal fear and anxiety, and specific stressors from unique child and maternal characteristics (medical complications, unusually difficult to care for child, maternal medical/mental health concerns) all contribute to differences in how a mother of an ill infant perceives her child and interacts with the youngster. These differences are most evident in the months following a child's birth, although observable differences in maternal interaction behaviors may persist to 1 year or slightly beyond (Crawford, 1982).

The relationship between early patterns of response in an infant and the mother's reactions to the infant's behaviors is significant for the development of communication skills. As has been noted, the primary developmental domain that differentiates healthy from ill infants is that of communicative development and performance. Hence, a continuum of risk must be adopted by the EI. To some degree, developmental delay (communication delay) does not appear or begin when the child does not use its first word at 1 year of age. The seeds to communication delay begin much earlier for many children. The communication delay observed in a majority of at-risk infants begins when proper patterns of attachment and interaction do not form. The process of inadequate attachment and interaction originates shortly after birth and is influenced by the child's medical condition and the mother's lack of access and caretaking opportunity. Information to be presented in later chapters furnishes suggestions for facilitating attachment and interaction, thereby increasing the potential for more normal patterns of communication to ensue.

Caregiver Response to a Medically Fragile Infant

Even under the best of circumstances, the birth of an infant, especially a firstborn infant, is a time of enormous change for parents—much more so in the case of a medically fragile infant. A review of the case studies provided at the outset of this chapter acquaints readers with the powerful set of responses and necessary adjustments set in motion when a child is born ill. Of necessity, the bulk of concern in the early days is directed toward the child, who is literally fighting for his or her life. However, the EI should be cognizant of the concurrent struggle that is taking place for the parents. It has been only recently that full attention has been directed toward the singular struggle that parents of at-risk infants face. It was previously suggested that anything the EI can do to enhance caregiver involvement in the intervention process benefits a child. Perhaps the first step in enhancing caregiver involvement is for the EI to gain a more complete understanding of the emotional barriers and adjustments that the parents face.

When children are born at risk, ill, or disabled, they are in need of physical and personal attention from an array of individuals. Not the least of these is the parents. Although the specific circumstances vary from child to child, new and unique demands are placed on the parents. In most instances, caregivers have never faced a similar set of circumstances. They are overwhelmed and fearful. These feelings may persist for a prolonged time. Refer back to the first case study presented in this chapter. The situation that Mark and Jan faced was compounded because they had two infants in need of special care. Although only one of their sons survived, Mark and Jan faced significant adjustments to the death of one son and the ongoing need for care of the surviving twin. Parents must adapt to a set of circumstances that are difficult and uncertain. Some parents adapt well, with others displaying a long-term pattern of behavior suggestive of incomplete adjustment. What is known about the distinctive adjustments parents of at-risk infants face? The material that follows informs the EI about these singular and complex adjustments.

EARLY ADJUSTMENTS

The first set of adjustments that parents must face revolves around the initial shock of having a premature, ill, or disabled child. When a woman gives birth to an ill infant, what changes in lifestyle is she likely to face? Her ability to make necessary adjustments may, in part, be related to her expectations prior to the birth of her special needs child. A review of the literature on mother's expectations before the birth of their children suggests that maternal experiences for the first several weeks following birth differ significantly from expectations. Gennaro, Grisemer, and Musci (1992) describe maternal reports following the birth of healthy children. The mothers reported spending less time than expected doing household chores, being with their husbands, having time for themselves, and engaging in recreational activities. Results suggested that mothers' expectations are different than their actual experiences during the first few weeks following a child's birth. Not having the healthy infant that mothers hope for adds a significant source of stress that must be addressed if full caregiver participation in early intervention is to be expected.

One important contribution to understanding the issues faced by parents of ill infants is provided by Taylor and Hall (1979). They point out that parents lose much when their child is born early or at risk, regardless of the cause. The psychological work that goes on during the later stages of pregnancy is important. Being deprived of those last weeks increases parental frustration following a child's preterm birth. When a child is born early or ill, unexpected reality replaces anticipated routines. Hence, the gap between parental expectation and actual circumstances is wide and perplexing. Taylor and Hall point out several stark adjustments that must be made by such parents.

First, a fragile, small, sick, and at-risk infant who is seriously ill or likely to become so, replaces the expected full-term infant. The initial shock is powerful and cannot be underestimated by the EI. Nurses frequently report that parents, on their first visit to the intensive care nursery and when seeing their child for the first time express a desire to turn away. In addition, parents show a reluctance to touch their newborn. This response is quite unlike that described earlier, in which parents are motivated to make physical contact with their child. An initial aversion to touch is prompted in large measure by fear and generally does not last for a long period of time.

Second, an unresponsive infant replaces the responsive baby they anticipated. Mothers of newborns are motivated to make initial contact with their offspring. In healthy situations, the baby responds to adult attempts to make contact. If the child is ill, it is unable to respond. Hence, early interaction and face-to-face contact and interchange are not possible. This is an important window of opportunity for the process of attachment and interaction to begin.

Third, the mother anticipated unrestricted, close, and frequent contact with her baby. This is not possible for the sick or disabled child. Rather than access, separation becomes the norm. This separation, depending on how long it lasts and maternal opportunity to provide some degree of caregiving, may result in the mother feeling that her child is a "stranger" to her. Lack of early contact and caregiving opportunity results in the mother and baby not getting to "know" one another.

The fourth aspect of parental adjustment is that, in many instances, parental expectations of caring for the baby in the comfort of their home is replaced by care provided in a hospital environment. Sophisticated and confusing equipment and routine replace the simplicity of a baby's crib beside the mother's bed in her home. She is unfamiliar with the routine, the equipment, and with what is expected of her (if anything) in this confusing and serious environment.

Maternal expectations included her functioning as the child's primary caregiver. Now she has been replaced by doctors and nurses who provide round-the-clock care for her baby. Although the care the child is provided is of high quality, the fact that it is being provided by a stranger is troublesome to her. Over time, the result may be a relinquishing of parental authority to these professional caregivers. She may face a need to reinvest herself as primary caregiver at a later date. In some instances, this is not a smooth and seamless transition.

Maternal attachment to the baby during the pregnancy was discussed previously in this chapter. Recall that the mother has, toward the end of the pregnancy, developed a set of expectations regarding her baby. Now she must face the fact that she has not produced the baby she expected. Her sense of failure may be acute. This results in a significant loss of self-esteem. Depending on her access to needed help, individual adjustment ability, and the child's immediate and later responses to her, this loss of self-esteem may prove to be a significant barrier to the formation of later attachment. Table 2–3 outlines parents' usual emotional reactions and adjustments to full-term and premature births. Overall, the mother rides an emotional roller coaster during the weeks and months following the birth of a premature or ill infant. The EI is encouraged to become familiar with these parental reactions as attempts to assist caregivers are made.

ONGOING ADJUSTMENTS

Parents face ongoing adjustments during and following periods of prolonged hospitalization for sick children. Most pediatric intensive care and neonatal intensive care units have made significant strides in addressing the weighty needs parents face during the ongoing stress that results. Support for families of children who are critically ill is provided by social workers, clergy, psychologists, psychiatrists, specially trained hospital staff, nurses, and doctors. Most recently, professionals have learned to let parents "tell us" what they need during these anxious times. Bass (1991) has provided data suggesting that parents are quite able to identify their most pressing needs during the period when their child is critically ill. Table 2–4 presents parental rat-

TABLE 2-3 Parents' Usual Emotional Reactions and Adjustments to Full-Term and Premature Births

	Full-Term	Preterm
Perception of events	Gain, success	Loss, failure
Reactions to birth	Joy, relief	Grief, concern
Emotional preparation	Complete	Incomplete
Expectations	Wished for baby	Feared baby
Self-esteem	Increased	Decreased
Baby's caregivers	Mother, father	Nurse, doctor
Parents and infants	Together	Separated
Baby's social responsiveness	Well developed	Absent
Mother goes home with:	Baby	Empty arms
Tasks remaining	Reconciling real baby and fantasized baby	Grieving for expected baby, anticipatory grieving for baby, accepting baby

Adapted from "Parent Infant Bonding: Problems and Opportunities in a Perinatal Center," by P. Taylor and B. Hall, 1979, *Seminars in Perinatology, 8*, p. 78.

TABLE 2-4 Parent Rating: Importance of Needs

Category	Mean Rating
Information	5.0
Attachment/parenting	5.0
Staff support	4.8
Child care	4.6
Physical support	4.3
Spiritual support	4.3

5 = extremely important;

4 = important;

3 = somewhat important;

2 = not very important;

1 = not important at all

Adapted from "What Do Parents Need When Their Infant Is a Patient in the NICU?" by L. Bass, 1991, *Neonatal Network, 10*, p. 25.

ings of need during their child's hospitalization. As may be observed, parents rate as extremely important their need for accurate information. In addition, they further indicate that they need assistance with attachment/parenting issues. Both of these needs, rated as extremely important, involve effective communication between parents and the professionals involved in providing care for their child. Additional information may be supplied by the EI who is involved in parent training, ongoing child follow-up, and intervention activities.

Trout and Foley (1989) list several sources of ongoing difficulty as parents adjust to the reality that their child presents them with new and uncertain challenges. The first area relates to parental confusion. Parents are often disappointed, angry, confused, and lonely. Parents may be able to verbalize these feelings. However, some parents are unaware that these feelings exist. Rather, their discomfort is expressed in other ways. A lack of pleasure while caring for their baby may result. They may feel that it is not pleasant to provide routine care. This may engender guilt on their part. The EI may be capable of helping parents identify and express these feelings and assist as they seek a better pattern of interaction and caretaking. Second, parents struggle with a sense of loss. After all, they have failed to produce the child they anticipated. They have lost self-esteem, control over their life, and freedom from worry that would not be there if their infant was healthy. Third, parents may be plagued by guilt. Guilt may interfere with full acceptance of the child. As one parent recently expressed, "Guilt is my constant companion." Fourth, parents are engaged in a continuous struggle to obtain and interpret the barrage of information they are exposed to. This information deluge begins when the child is hospitalized and continues for a long time. Information emerges related to short- and long-term issues. Parents are provided with information from a variety of sources. Some of it is communicated well, with other information communicated poorly, leading to further confusion. Some professionals communicate effectively and with compassion and understanding. Other professionals communicate in an impersonal and detached manner that does not convey acceptance to the parents. Finally, as Trout and Foley (1989) note, overall family dynamics are upset when a disabled child is taken home. Siblings may resent their sick brother or sister. The child becomes the focus of attention. Older children may not have an effective and available means of expressing their true feelings. Overall family routine is disrupted. Family schedules, patterns of communication, activities, and general equilibrium are upset. The EI must not overlook these substantial issues.

The term "chronic sorrow" has been used to describe the ongoing range of adjustments that parents of special needs children face. The resurgence of grief, loss, guilt, and fear during stressor events in the child's life (illness, developmental crises, change) cannot be overlooked by the EI. It has also been noted that mothers and fathers differ in the manner in which they view the child immediately after birth and over time as ongoing crises arise. Hummel and Eastman (1991) investigated the range of feelings that surface after the birth of a preterm infant. The difficulties that parents of preterm infants face are not unlike those faced by parents of older special needs children. Table 2–5 lists these feelings. What is readily noted are the instances in which there are significant differences between mothers' and fathers' frequency of "yes" answers. Such information is of immeasurable help to the EI interested in enhancing caregivers' adjustment to the set of circumstances they face.

Table 2–6 identifies the percentage of parents who answer "yes" about the presence of various feelings during ongoing stressor events.

TABLE 2-5   Parental Feelings Following Preterm Birth

Percentage of Yes Answers*			
Feelings	All Parents	Mothers	Fathers
Shock	59	68	48
Frustration	66	75	53
Fear of leaving child	56	69	39
Emptiness	53	68	34
Depression	51	64	34
Hurt	50	66	30
Crying easily	50	78	14
Irritability	47	61	27
Sleep difficulties	45	59	25
Anger	44	59	25
Self-blame	36	58	27
Self-pity	24	32	14
Feelings of isolation	23	37	25
Wanting to be alone	17	25	25

*All differences between mothers and fathers are at the p < .05 or better level.

Adapted from "Do Parents of Preterm Infants Suffer Chronic Sorrow?" by P. Hummel and D. Eastman, 1991, *Neonatal Network, 10*, p. 59.

TABLE 2-6   Parental Feelings with Stressor Events

Stressful Experience	Feelings	Percentage of Yes Answers
Illness	Helplessness	64
	Thinking about child continually	53
	Frustration	52
	Fear child may die	51
Surgery	Helplessness	74
	Thinking about child continually	71
	Fear child may die	71
	Fear of future	58
	Frustration	52
Developmental delay	Fear of abnormal development	57
	Fear of other problems	47
Behavior problems	Frustration	33
	Fear of inability to handle problems	33

Adapted from "Do Parents of Preterm Infants Suffer Chronic Sorrow?" by P. Hummel and D. Eastman, 1991, *Neonatal Network*, *10*, p. 59.

Again, this is information that the EI should use in all interactions with parents. It is also valuable to note that although parents may be adjusting to the special needs they face together, their individual perceptions may differ markedly. As the EI interacts with parents, it must be recalled that there are literally three babies under discussion: his, hers, and the EI's. It is the EI's responsibility to assist the caregivers to see the same baby.

A final comment about ongoing issues faced by parents of ill infants relates to the increased risk of abuse and neglect. Although reports vary somewhat, an increased incidence of abuse is observed in children with a history of premature delivery, low birth weight, and illness during infancy. Although predisposition to abuse/neglect may exist before the birth of a child, the adjustment issues outlined above may serve to decrease attachment and interaction, thereby increasing the potential for parenting disorders (abuse/neglect). Abused children are known to be characterized as younger aged (infants and young children), male, low birth weight, premature, frequently ill, neurologically impaired (mild), and developmentally delayed. These represent child-related preabuse characteristics (Williams, 1978).

PARENT-PROFESSIONAL COMMUNICATION

Anything that the EI can do to enhance caregiver involvement in the early intervention process is important. The material just presented describes the variety of issues that parents face when attempting to establish optimal patterns of attachment and interaction. It is imperative that the EI keep in mind the immediate and long-term issues parents face.

In addition to the concerns already expressed, it is interesting to note that an added barrier to caregiver involvement in early intervention may be the nature of the relationship that exists between the caregiver and the EI.

If the EI is concerned about facilitating full caregiver participation in intervention, understanding barriers that can exist between the EI and parents is imperative. Stonestreet, Johnson, and Acton (1991) describe the results of an investigation designed to determine the nature of these barriers. The results of this investigation identify several comments parents frequently make about interventionists and additional comments EIs make about parents.

What Parents Say about Interventionists

Interventionists don't listen to us. Parents make this their number one observation. Parental observations include the impression that, in many instances, professionals involved in service provision already have their mind made up. Parents express the opinion that interventionists are not really interested in what they have to say.

Interventionists don't take time with us. Parents consistently express frustration related to the amount of control the interventionist has over the amount of time spent with parents. Conferences are felt to be too short, with important decisions about the child made to fit into an allotted time frame.

Interventionists talk in strange ways. Parents are continually dumfounded by the vocabulary used to describe their child. Professional jargon abounds. Parents may feel the jargon used by the EI is a way of reminding them who is in charge.

Interventionists don't answer our questions. Simple answers to direct questions are what parents desire. Continual referral to other professionals for answers is frustrating to parents. A simple "I don't know" may be the best response the EI can provide.

Interventionists don't guess why. Although attaching labels to children is a difficult process for the interventionist, many parents express frustration unless the EI is willing to provide cause-and-effect information. Caregivers are willing to accept the EI's "best guess" about causation. The EI should inform the parents that their "guess" may need modification over time and as new information about the child becomes available.

Interventionists keep information from us. Parents frequently operate under the general assumption that the EI tells them what they think parents should know but that additional information is withheld.

Interventionists don't ask for our opinion. Parents' frustration is increased if they believe that important decisions are made without their input. The EI may spend considerable time trying to convince parents that a particular decision is best for the child. However, comparable time may not be spent in allowing the parents to fully express their opinions.

What Interventionists Say about Today's Parents

Parents don't answer our questions. Many interventionists indicate that they feel that the information they receive from parents, especially for children under 3 years of age, lacks candor. There may be a variety of reasons why caregivers are reluctant to fully answer the EI's questions. Whatever the cause, the EI needs accurate and reliable information to provide comprehensive services to children.

Parents don't take time to help us. Consistent frustration is noted by EIs when parents do not follow suggested intervention activities. Missing conferences, inconsistent administration of prescribed medication, lack of follow-through on home programs, lack of consistency if assistive devices are needed (hearing aids, and so on), and general lack of dependability in various areas of caregiver responsibility are reported.

Parents don't listen to us. Many interventionists feel that parents have their mind made up and will not accept input from the EI team. The feeling that parents hear only what they want to hear is frequently reported by EIs.

Parents keep information from us. Parents of children at home spend much more time with the child than does the EI. Hence, new behaviors, indications of progress, and other sources of new information are vital to the EI. Many EIs feel that parents are not consistent in informing them of information of this nature.

Parents insist that we make the decisions. The EI desires caregiver involvement in decision making. In many instances, however, the EI is put in the position of being mostly responsible for important intervention decisions. Comments such as "You are the teacher, do what you think best" are common.

Parents don't agree on child behavior. Lack of agreement between parents when describing child behaviors can be a source of confusion for the EI. The EI should not be put in the position of deciding who (mother or father) is right in providing important information.

Parents guess on diagnosis. Parents often provide guesses as to why their child is in need of intervention services. These guesses may be based on partial truth gained from the media, friends, other parents, or something they have read but do not fully understand. Parents may waste time and energy by continually trying to "guess" about the nature of their child's difficulty.

Parents talk in strange ways. Parents frequently stray from the topic, do not provide direct answers to questions, and in other ways do not communicate effectively with early intervention professionals. This is a source of frustration for the EI.

Additional information contained in the Stonestreet et al. (1991) article provides information designed to assist the EI in establishing effective communication with parents. These suggestions are presented in Table 2–7. The EI can be quite active in reducing parental feelings of distance and estrangement by implementing simple and common sense strategies. The result is to reduce caregivers' feelings of not being full members of the team, thereby making their overall adjustment more successful.

SUMMARY OF PARENTAL ADJUSTMENT DIFFICULTIES

Information presented thus far has demonstrated that both the infant and the caregiver face significant hurdles in establishing optimal patterns of interaction and attachment. The infant's illness, caregiver adjustments (short- and long-term), the nature of the intensive care nursery, parental anxiety, and communication problems with interventionists may serve to distance parents from their child and the intervention process. Distancing from the intervention process has its

TABLE 2-7 Interventionist Suggestions for Enhancing Caregiver-Interventionist Communication

● Create an atmosphere of exchange	● Facilitate parent participation in the intervention process
● Recognize specific needs of particular parents	● Refrain from using excessive jargon
● Furnish necessary information	● Be sensitive to the ongoing grieving process
● Ensure parental feelings of success	● Recognize parents' need for peer support
● Develop active listening skills	● Make parents full participants in planning
● Provide legitimate program options	● Focus on outcomes

Adapted from "Guidelines for Real Partnerships With Parents," by R. Stonestreet, R. Johnson, and S. Acton, 1991, *Infant Toddler Intervention, 1,* p. 37.

roots in the patterns of deficient attachment and interaction discussed thus far.

Parents frequently report that their primary feeling when they are allowed to take their child home from the hospital is one of anger. Although they are quite anxious about the lifestyle changes they face, their anger is difficult to deal with and may become a barrier to full participation in the intervention process. In addition to anger, caregivers report that during the course of hospitalization and immediately following the transition home, they are left with three distinct impressions.

First, they may be made to feel "dumb." This is communicated to them through lack of communication while the child is hospitalized. Their impression is that the medical staff withholds information or does not fully answer questions because the parents will not be able to understand it. Parents are not allowed access to the child's medical chart. Even if they are allowed to read the chart, much of what it contains is confusing to them. Recall that parents expressed that their primary need was for information. This may not be routinely provided for them.

Second, they feel "dangerous." Throughout the child's hospitalization, restrictions are placed on the amount of touch allowed and their opportunity to provide care. Parents are cautioned about the equipment in the NICU and their need to reduce noise and overall stimulation. Over time, parents may form the distinct impression that they are in the way and perhaps even dangerous.

Third, they feel "disenfranchised." For varying amounts of time, routine care of their child is provided by someone else. They may begin to feel that they are not part of the general process taking place. As control is relinquished to others, they become spectators. Franchising them may become difficult and the transition to their functioning as primary caregivers may not be a smooth one.

These are significant issues. Hence, it is imperative that the EI be involved in activities designed to enhance caregiver attachment and interaction. The result may be better participation in early intervention and improved communication skills for the child.

ENHANCING CAREGIVER-INFANT ATTACHMENT AND INTERACTION

An initial step in improving maternal-infant interaction/attachment and parental participation in the early intervention process is to increase caregiver feelings of "investment." Recall that the nature of the process for ill infants distances the caregiver. Hence, once the child transitions home, the caregiver may feel that he or she is taking a stranger home. Directing attention toward preventing caregiver distancing at the earliest stages, rather than at a later date, appears most logical. Strategies designed to enhance attachment while the child is hospitalized and following discharge to the home, plus the efficacy of such activities, are discussed next.

Parent Support Groups

Support groups are not a new phenomenon. It has been more recently that the concept of support groups has been applied to parents whose children are hospitalized. Many intensive care nurseries throughout the United States and the rest of the world provide parent support groups. Groups of this nature take a variety of forms. Some are led by parents, some are led by the hospital staff, others are organized by mental health professionals, while additional groups are initiated by the clergy. Whatever the nature of a group, support of this nature is quite helpful to caregivers who are struggling with the adjustments delineated throughout this chapter. The EI may be able to initiate or participate in parent support groups.

One promising parent support group model is provided by Scott and Doyle (1985). This model offers a one-to-one match between new parents and trained parents who have a disabled or at-risk child at home. The contact between the new parents and the trained parent takes place as soon as possible. The "helping parents" meet with the new parents and encourage them to become part of a small group of parents who are undergoing similar experiences. Although small groups of this nature may initially lack structure, a variety of issues may be dealt with. Parents who participate in groups of this nature report a decreased sense of isolation, greater access to helpful information, and a general cathartic effect due to shared experiences with other group members. An additional parent-to-parent program is described by Lindsay et al. (1993). In this parent support program, a professional program coordinator recruited and trained volunteer parents with past experience with sick infants. These volunteers provided support for new parents through hospital visits, phone contacts, and home visits during the child's first year of life. Three broad areas of support were identified. These were emotional support, informational support, and maternal role support. The Lindsay et al. investigation employed an experimental and a control group. Significant differences between groups were found on measures of maternal mood states, maternal-infant relationships, and home environment. Mothers receiving parent-to-parent support reported better maternal mood states, including less anger, depression, and anxiety, than did mothers who were not receiving support. In addition, treatment mothers had better maternal-infant relationships, and better home environments 12 months after hospital discharge, than did the comparison group of mothers.

One carefully controlled study on the efficacy of support groups was conducted by Minde et al. (1980). This investigation used both a control and an experimental group. Infants and parents were matched on all important variables. The experimental group parents received group support and the control group did not. The focus of the group was to provide parents with a forum in which they could talk about and learn to cope with the stresses they faced with having an ill child. The group also attempted to assist parents in learning how to cope with the highly technical routines and procedures employed in the hospital and how to handle interactions with many different professionals. Finally, the group was designed to help parents obtain adequate information from appropriate medical personnel, to recognize and meet present and future needs of their child, and to utilize supportive community resources following hospital discharge. Table 2–8 summarizes some of the findings of the study. As may be observed, the mothers who were part of a group scored significantly higher on measures related to understanding their child's

TABLE 2-8 Comparison of Control and Experimental Groups: Effects of Parental Support Groups

Measure	Control	Experimental	Significance
Satisfaction with information	3.5	4.4	<.01
Understanding of infant's condition	2.8	3.8	<.01
Interaction with other parents	2.0	3.8	<.01
Comfort with ability to provide care at home	3.1	3.8	<.05
Knowledge of community resources	2.7	3.9	<.001
Total scores	22.1	28.7	<.001

Adapted from "Self-Help Groups in a Premature Nursery: A Controlled Evaluation," by K. Minde, N. Shosenberg, P. Marton, J. Thompson, J. Ripley, and S. Burns, 1980, *The Journal of Pediatrics*, *96*, p. 933.

condition, interaction with other parents, level of comfort with ability to care for infant following discharge, frequency of hospital visits, and knowledge of community resources. In addition, the mothers in the experimental group interacted with their children to a greater degree. Several of these differences were observed up to 3 months postdischarge from the hospital, the point at which follow-up ceased.

Although empirical support for parent support groups is still emerging, the investigations mentioned provide promising results. The EI is encouraged to facilitate the concept of parent support groups regardless of the EI's employment setting or the population of children with disabilities worked with.

Caregiver Education

Caregivers rate their desire for accurate, reliable, and helpful information following the birth of an ill child (Bass, 1991) as extremely important. Hence, the EI is encouraged to become familiar with a broad array of material that may be communicated to caregivers. Regardless of their employment setting, EIs are in a unique position to convey needed information to parents. The result will be improved communication and enhanced parental participation in intervention activities. The material to follow is designed to demonstrate that timely information provided to the parents will result in increased caregiver-child interaction and greater parental involvement in the intervention process.

Teaching mothers about the abilities of their newborns may facilitate early attachment, interaction, and participation in intervention activities (Meisels, Jones, & Stiefel, 1983). Instruction of this nature has taken a variety of forms and has been provided by professionals in various fields. The information communicated to parents may relate to concerns regarding medical, developmental, financial, parenting, attachment, family, and long-term expectations. These are important matters for parents, with their need for information being substantial.

Investigations designed to monitor the effectiveness of parent-oriented training on child and parent measures have been conducted by Nurcome et al. (1984) and Widmayer and Field (1980, 1981). Long- and short-term measures were made. These studies suggest that mother-only training is not sufficient to make significant changes in an infant's developmental profile. However, enduring effects on the parents were noted. These studies suggest that educating parents on how to perceive infant behavioral states and cues, handling and positioning, feeding, and social capabilities does make a difference for the parents.

Pokorni, Osborn, and Aldrich (1992) describe a program of in-service education provided for NICU staff. Although the information was originally designed to alert hospital personnel to caregiving issues for ill infants, the information is readily applicable to parents. The content of the in-service video covered material related to premature development, the NICU environment, positioning and handling of the child, the growing preemie, and family-related issues. A pre-post assessment indicated that those who received the in-service instruction significantly improved their information base about the issues covered. A similar study is reported by L. Harrison, Sherrod, Dunn, Olivet, and Jeong (1992). This investigation measured parental ability to accurately monitor their child's interactions. Instruction provided to the parents included a description of behavioral cues in infants and unique infant characteristics. Mothers who received this training were better able to rate their child's behaviors than those who did not.

A different approach toward measuring the effectiveness of parental education is reported by Saylor, Elksnin, Farah, and Pope (1990). This investigation was designed to assess professionals' ratings of the effectiveness of various procedures designed to maximize parental participation in early intervention. Table 2–9 summarizes the results using a rating scale of 1 to 5 (1 = not at all successful, 5 = completely successful). As may be observed, providing information to par-

TABLE 2–9 Professionals' Ratings Regarding Maximizing Caregiver Involvement in Early Intervention

Procedure	Likely Effectiveness
Information packet	3.4
Names/phone numbers of staff	3.3
Information on child development	3.5
Audiovisual aids	3.9
Information library	3.4

Note: Ratings on a 5-point scale from (5) completely successful to (1) not at all successful.

Adapted from "Depends on Who You Ask: What Maximizes Participation of Families in Early Intervention Programs," by C. Saylor, N. Elksnin, B. Farah, and J. Pope, 1990, *Journal of Pediatric Psychology*, *15*, p. 557.

ents rated between 3.4 and 3.8 for likely effectiveness. This is as high or higher than any other strategies surveyed by the investigators.

Caregivers' need for information is regularly reported in the literature on early intervention. Various strategies to provide this information have proven to be effective. Overall, anything the EI can do to provide accurate, timely, and reliable information for caregivers adjusting to the changes they face following the birth of an ill child should serve to enhance caregiver-infant attachment and interaction, as well as parent participation in the early intervention process.

Caregiver Responsibility during Hospitalization

One of the most powerful influences in reducing attachment and interaction, thereby affecting caregiver involvement in later intervention, is the lack of opportunity afforded caregivers to provide care while the child is ill. Although significant change has taken place in recent years, many parents continue to report that they feel "in the way" during periods of prolonged hospitalization. Over time, this impression increases their feelings of disenfranchisement as parents. The result may be less-than-optimal participation in ongoing intervention activities.

One of the most effective strategies the EI, regardless of primary academic discipline, can encourage is to put parents to work. Said in another way, parents should be allowed much greater involvement in the provision of ongoing care for their sick child. This may take a variety of forms and depends on parental level of comfort, training, staff comfort, and hospital routine. Several suggestions are listed in the following material.

Charting

Copious and detailed paperwork is kept for children during hospitalization. Parents should be allowed to participate in providing information for the child's medical chart. The caregiver should be allowed access to the child's chart for such purposes. At the very least, the caregiver should be provided with an additional chart. The exact nature of the information parents provide on the chart may vary. The important aspect of this suggestion is not the content of the parents' chart, but rather that they are involved in providing care. Involvement of this nature changes them from passive observers to involved participants. Even during times when the child is critically ill and does not show awareness of the parents' presence, assigning responsibility to the parents in the form of charting makes them feel part of the process and lessens their feelings of being "dangerous." The content of parental charting may vary. Parents may be asked to provide information relative to the child's weight (daily measures), respiratory performance, nutritional intake, medical and nonmedical interventions (what/when/who), wake-sleep cycles, medications administered, special procedures, daily schedule of activities, consultations, level of alertness, and interaction cues. Although each hospital may have restrictions on parental involvement of this nature (direct input by nonmedical staff on the child's permanent hospital chart), there should be no objection to providing a separate chart for parents. The cost is minimal, little additional effort is needed on the part of hospital staff, and the benefit to parents may be substantial.

One strategy that affords parents an opportunity to collect ongoing data regarding their child is to involve them in structuring the child's developmental care plan. Caregiver involvement in this manner requires that the caregivers provide input and ongoing monitoring of overall changes in the child's condition during hospitalization. One positive aspect of this strategy is that as the child's behavioral responses change over time, the caregiver must become alert to these changes and communicate them to the staff and others. As the child gains greater physiological stability, interaction with caregivers will change. Parents will benefit greatly from increased ability to note these changes and will feel less "in the way."

Caregiving

The majority of touch that takes place in the hospital is medical in nature. In addition, those infants who might benefit from more interaction with adults generally receive less attention. Greater detail relative to touch will be provided in later chapters. However, attempts should be made to allow parents increased opportunity to care for the child. This may involve a variety of activities.

Feeding becomes a major concern for ill infants. Nutritional support is essential for a child to gain weight and for general physiologic stability. A variety of professionals are directing attention to improvement of feeding and swallowing for sick infants. Parents are involved in these activities to varying degrees. From the beginning, parents should be an important part of all feeding activities. Following hospital discharge, parents report that feeding is a major source of frustration for them. Parental involvement from the earliest attempts at feeding may serve to reduce this frustration. In addition, early involvement in feeding gives parents a sense of accomplishment and franchisement in the child's care.

Infection control is a major issue in hospitals. Bathing the child, changing diapers and linens, and rotating disposable equipment are regular activities that parents may perform. In general, greater access to the child and involvement in the care of the child within the bounds dictated by the child's medical condition are suggested. In the past, physical separation of parents from infants was the norm. More recently, parents are provided with greater access to their child. Unrestricted visiting is allowed in many NICUs. In NICUs that have allowed increased parental involvement, positive effects have been noted. Increased parental access to their ill infant has resulted in greater parental interest in the child. The difference between limited versus unlimited parental access and involvement in the hospital has been noted by several investigators. In NICUs that allow unlimited access, only 2.2% of mothers fail to interact with the child, whereas 13% of mothers fail to interact if limited access is afforded them. Furthermore, when the baby is in the crib, mothers who have been previously allowed unlimited access interact with their child more and display fewer negative feelings. Increased access and involvement in caregiving increase parental feelings of involvement, interest, and interaction (Paludetto, Perfetto, Aspera, DeCurtis, & Paludetto, 1981). Additional caretaking activities, such as kangaroo care and participation in medical interventions, enhance caretaking as well. During one recent visit to a NICU, the author observed a physician performing a minor surgical procedure on an infant. One of the people assisting the physician was the infant's mother. She had scrubbed and dressed in appropriate sterile clothing, was wearing rubber gloves and mask, and was actually handing the physician the appropriate surgical instruments under the direction of a nurse. This is a powerful example of how caregivers may assist in actual caregiving during initial hospitalization.

Decision Making

One area in which parents have traditionally been allowed only minimal participation is that of decision making. Without a doubt, difficult decisions must be made on a variety of issues that parents of ill children face. Across the United States and internationally, there are significant differences in the degree to which parents are involved in decision making while a child is hospitalized. These differences stem from hospital practice, physician judgment, parental willingness to be involved, and the condition of the child (relative to short- and long-term issues). In large measure, parents are hostage to a set of circumstances that they cannot control. H. Harrison (1986) notes that physicians discuss among themselves decisions that must be made but that parents are rarely involved in these decisions. The question of how fully parents should be involved in decision making is not within the scope of this chapter. However, the sense of powerlessness voiced by many parents can be reduced as caregivers are afforded greater access and involvement in the decision-making process. Parents report that they feel responsible for the child, yet at the same time are not granted authority in decision making. The EI is encouraged, as far as possible, to provide accurate information to parents and to engage them in discussions relative to a host of decisions that must be made as the time nears for a child to be released from the hospital. One manner in which caregivers can feel less alienated from their child, thereby enhancing their participation in the intervention process, is to actively engage them in discussions about all aspects of their child's care dealing with short- and long-term issues.

The Transition Home

Each year, thousands of children with special needs move from the hospital to the home or from one intervention service setting to another. The issues raised thus far in this chapter point out the increased risk for lack of full caregiver participation in the early intervention process. Certainly, additional attention must be directed toward a very important time for the child and the family: the period when the child transitions home and the parents become primary caregivers. Rosenkoetter, Hains, and Fowler (1994) point out that transitions constitute a critical point during which the early interventionist can have an important impact. In a discussion of what is known about transitions, the authors note several factors.

First, all children, regardless of age or disability, face transitions. They cannot be avoided. Children and families who enter early childhood intervention programs must eventually move from one setting to another. The EI can be instrumental in alerting parents to the transitions they face as a child passes through the intervention process.

Second, early transitions are very important. The transition home from the hospital, the transition into a new intervention setting, or general changes in the family that affect the intervention being provided at any given time are significant. This is particularly true for caregivers who are dealing with significant adjustment issues related to the need for them to assume the role of primary caregivers.

Parents must also be reminded that transitions inevitably involve change of one type or another. This can be stressful. Changes may involve new interventionists, new settings, new materials, new goals for the child, and even new terms used to describe the child's performance and future expectations. During times of change, caregivers must be reminded that they are the constant in the child's life. Everything else may change over time, but their involvement must remain constant. Change can be stressful for anyone and particularly so for the parents of a special needs child. As Rosenkoetter et al. (1994) suggest, one key to effective transitions is caregiver education and participation in planning. The EI can play an integral role in making transitions less stressful. Additional information on the transition from the hospital to the home setting is provided in several investigations (Barker, 1991; Katz, 1993; Robinson, 1991). Barker lists several areas in which parents display struggle as hospital discharge approaches. These are summarized in Table 2–10. These issues are significant for the caregiver. The EI can have an important impact in assisting caregivers in the transition to the home setting in light of the information presented in this table.

Additional assistance in transition planning is provided by Katz (1993). Project Headed Home targets three major areas. These include the family of the ill child, the child, and the medical and nursing staff. Project activities, in the context of making the passage home less stressful, include several steps. First, a determination of the family's resources and major concerns must be made. Following this, parents are provided with instruction designed to develop their sense of competence in self-management of the child's medical and developmental needs. This instruction translates into facilitating the caregivers' ability to incorporate developmental activities into routine care activities

TABLE 2-10   The Transition Home

- Parents feel ambivalence prior to discharge
- They are uncertain about the child's impact upon the family
- They have significant fears about their competence to meet the child's needs
- They do not understand the child's vulnerability
- They are fearful about their ability to adequately feed the child
- They struggle with the short- and long-term impact of prematurity on the child's health and development

Adapted from Barker, A. (1991).

in the hospital and home. Finally, the parents are provided with information about community resources and their need to advocate for additional services the child needs. This approach appears to provide parents with a broad base of information, thus preparing them for the new set of issues they face once they become responsible for full care of their child in the home setting.

Robinson (1991) provides additional information on the transition home. An important factor in the information provided by Robinson is on incorporation of hospital discharge planning into a child's overall care plan. This approach changes planning of this nature from an afterthought into an integral part of the child's overall plan. Robinson suggests the importance of effective assessment of the home environment, specific discharge teaching goals, and inclusion of significant others into the transition process. What emerges from strategies such as these is the distinct impression that the EI can have an effective role in making a move home less stressful and uncertain for parents. The result is less anxiety and improved participation in the intervention process.

CHAPTER SUMMARY

Perhaps the best way to highlight the importance of the issues raised in this chapter is to describe an experience the author had in a NICU. During a consultation provided in a large hospital in the Midwest, the author was asked to observe an infant who had been hospitalized for 10 weeks. The child was quite ill, having been 10 weeks premature, weighing 950 g at birth. Hospital records indicated that the infant was seriously hearing impaired, perhaps deaf, and had suffered a grade

IV intercranial hemorrhage. Further review of the medical chart indicated that significant visual damage was present, along with intermittent seizures and cardiac problems. In short, this child, a boy, was seriously ill with significant concerns relative to long-term developmental expectations. On the day of the consultation, the mother was visiting. Following examination of the child, the mother was asked by the neonatologist if she would like to hold the child. This was her first opportunity to hold her son.

The mother spoke no English, only Spanish. She sat in a rocker next to the child's bed as the physician reached in, picked up the child, and handed him to her. She held him for a few moments, started to sob, and then turned to the physician to ask a simple question. The question she asked was uncomplicated, yet penetrating and revealing. She asked twice, in Spanish, if it was "OK for me to kiss my baby."

Any clinician familiar with the environment of the NICU is forced to ask an equally powerful question in return. What had been communicated to that mother that led her to believe that she must ask for permission to perform the most basic of maternal responses toward her child? This is the environment in which at-risk and disabled infants and their parents live.

The purpose of this chapter is to point out that the birth and early experience of an ill infant are qualitatively different from those of a healthy child. These differences relate to issues of attachment, interaction, and caregiver adjustment. Living with children who require significant alteration in normal family routine affects families in varying degrees. The EI becomes a participant in this process as intervention services are initiated. For the EI to do all that is possible to enhance caregiver involvement in the intervention process, a full understanding of the concerns raised in this chapter is necessary. To fail to do so decreases the effectiveness of the services the EI delivers.

REFERENCES

Ali, Z., & Lowry, M. (1981). Early maternal-child contact: Effects on later behavior. *Developmental Medicine and Child Neurology, 23,* 337.

Als, H., & Brazelton, B. (1981). A new model of assessing behavioral organization in preterm and full-term infants: Two case studies. *Journal of the American Academy of Child Psychiatry, 20,* 239.

Bakeman, R., & Brown, J. (1977). An approach to the assessment of mother-infant interaction. *Child Development, 51,* 195.

Barker, A. (1991). The transition home for preterm infants. *Neonatal Network, 3,* 65.

Bass, L. (1991). What do parents need when their infant is a patient in the NICU? *Neonatal Network, 10,* 25.

Brazelton, T., & Cramer, B. (1990). *The earliest relationship.* Reading, MA: Addison-Wesley.

Brown, J., & Bakeman, R. (1980). Relationships of human mothers with their infants during the first year of life: Effects of prematurity. In R. Bell & W. Smotherman (Eds.), *Maternal influences and early behaviors* (p. 120). New York: Spectrum.

Crawford, J. (1982). Mother-infant interaction in premature and full-term infants. *Child Development, 53,* 957.

Field, T. (1977). Effects of early separation: Experimental manipulations of infant-mother face-to-face interactions. *Child Development, 48,* 763.

Field, T. (1980a). Interactions of high risk infants: Quantitative and qualitative differences. In D. Swain (Ed.), *Exceptional infant-psychosocial risks in infant-environment transactions.* New York: Bruner-Mazel.

Field, T. (1983). High risk infants have less fun during early interactions. *Topics in Early Childhood Special Education, 3,* 77.

Gennaro, S., Grisemer, A., & Musci, R. (1992). Expected versus actual lifestyle changes in mothers of preterm low birth weight children. *Neonatal Network, 11,* 39.

Goldberg, S. (1990). Attachment in infants: Theory, research, and practice. *Infants and Young Children, 2,* 11.

Goldson, E. (1992). The neonatal intensive care unit: Premature infants and parents. *Infants and Young Children, 4,* 31.

Harrison, H. (1986). Neonatal intensive care: Parents' role in ethical decision making. *Birth, 3,* 165.

Harrison, L. Sherrod, A., Dunn, L., Olivet, L., & Jeong, J. (1992). Effects of hospital based instruction on interactions between parents and preterm infants. *Neonatal Network, 9,* 27.

Hummel, P., & Eastman, D. (1991). Do parents of preterm infants suffer chronic sorrow? *Neonatal Network, 10,* 59.

Katz, K. (1993). Project headed home: Intervention in the pediatric intensive care unit for infants and their families. *Infants and Young Children, 5,* 67.

Klaus, M., & Fanaroff, A. (Eds.). (1979). *Care of the high risk neonate.* Philadelphia: W. B. Saunders.

Klaus, M., & Kennell, J. (1976). *Maternal-infant bonding.* St. Louis, MO: C. V. Mosby.

Klaus, M., Leger, T., & Trause, A. (Eds.). (1982). *Maternal attachment and mothering disorders.* Sausalito, CA: Johnson & Johnson.

Lindsay, J., Roman, L., De Wys, M., Eager, M., Levick, J., & Quinn, M. (1993). Creative caring in the NICU: Parent-to-parent support. *Neonatal Network, 12,* 37.

McFarlane, A. (1978). Maternal attachments. In S. Kitzinger & J. Davis (Eds.), *The place of birth* (p. 96). New York: Oxford University Press.

Meisels, S., Jones, S., & Stiefel, G. (1983). Neonatal intervention: Problem, purpose, and prospects. *Topics in Early Childhood Special Education, 3,* 1.

Minde, K. (1983). Effect of neonatal complications in premature infants on early parent-infant interactions. *Developmental Medicine and Child Neurology, 25,* 763.

Minde, K., Perotta, M., & Martin, P. (1985). Maternal caretaking and play with full-term and premature infants. *Journal of Child Psychiatry and Allied Disciplines, 26,* 231.

Minde, K., Shosenberg, N., Marton, P., Thompson, J., Ripley, J., & Burns, S. (1980). Self-help groups in a premature nursery—A controlled evaluation. *The Journal of Pediatrics, 96,* 933.

Nurcome, B., Howell, D., Rauh, V., Teti, D., Ruoff, P., & Brennan, J. (1984). An intervention program for mothers of low birthweight infants: Preliminary results. *Academy of Child Psychiatry, 23,* 319.

Oehler, J., Hannan, T., & Catlett, A. (1993). Maternal views of preterm infants' responsiveness to social interaction. *Neonatal Network, 12,* 67.

Paludetto, R., Perfetto, M., Aspera, A., DeCurtis, M., & Paludetto, M. (1981). Reactions of sixty parents allowed unrestricted contact with infants in the neonatal intensive care unit. *Early Human Development, 5,* 401.

Pederson, D. (1987). Maternal emotional responses to preterm birth. *American Journal of Orthopsychiatry, 57,* 15.

Pokorni, J., Osborn, D., & Aldrich, M. (1992). Using inservice videotapes to promote caregiving behaviors in the NICU. *Neonatal Network, 11,* 43.

Provence, S. (1990). Interactional issues: Infants, parents, professionals. *Infants and Young Children, 3,* 1.

Robinson, T. (1991). Discharge teaching in the NICU. *Neonatal Network, 10,* 77.

Rose, S. (1983). Behavioral and psychophysiological sequelae of preterm birth: The neonatal period. In T. Field & A. Sostek (Eds.), *Infants born at risk* (p. 258). New York: Grune & Stratton.

Rosenkoetter, S., Hains, A., & Fowler, S. (1994). *Bridging early services for children with special needs and their families.* Baltimore: Paul H. Brookes.

Ross, G. (1980). Parental responses to infants in intensive care: The separation issue reevaluated. In P. Auld (Ed.), *Clinics in Perinatology, 7,* 47.

Rossetti, L. (1990). *Infant-toddler assessment.* Austin, TX: PRO-ED.

Saylor, C., Elksnin, N., Farah, B., & Pope, J. (1990). Depends on who you ask: What maximizes participation of families in early intervention programs. *Journal of Pediatric Psychology, 15,* 557.

Scott, S., & Doyle, P. (1985). Parent-to-parent support. In M. Schleifer & S. Klein (Eds.), *The disabled child and the family: An exceptional parent reader* (p. 134). Boston: Exceptional Parent Press.

Sparks, S., Oas, M., & Erickson, R. (1988, November). *Clinical services to infants at risk for communication disorders.* Paper presented at the annual convention of the American Speech-Language-Hearing Association, Boston.

Stonestreet, R., Johnson, R., & Acton, S. (1991). Guidelines for real partnerships with parents. *Infant-Toddler Intervention, 1,* 37.

Taylor, P., & Hall, B. (1979). Parent-infant bonding: Problems and opportunities in a perinatal center. *Seminars in Perinatology, 3,* 73.

Trout, M., & Foley, G. (1989). Working with families of handicapped infants and toddlers. *Topics in Language Disorders, 10,* 57.

Widmayer, S., & Field, T. (1980). Effects of Brazelton demonstrations on early interactions of preterm infants and their teenage mothers. *Infant Behavior and Development, 3,* 79.

Widmayer, S., & Field, T. (1981). Effects of Brazelton demonstration for mothers on the development of preterm infants. *Pediatrics, 67,* 711.

Williams, G. (1978). Child abuse. In P. Magrab (Ed.), *Psychological management of pediatric problems* (p. 250). Baltimore: University Park Press.

Zarling, C., Hirsch, B., & Landry, S. (1988). Maternal social networks and mother-infant interactions in full-term and very low birthweight, preterm infants. *Child Development, 59,* 178.

CHAPTER

3

Assessment of Socio-Communicative Skills in Infants and Toddlers

❝ Assessment is any activity, either formal through the use of norm-referenced standardized criteria, or less formal, through the use of developmental profiles or checklists, that is designed to elicit accurate and reliable samples of behavior upon which inferences relative to developmental skill status may be made. ❞

Perhaps no activity challenges the skills of the early interventionist more than gaining accurate and reliable assessment results. Furthermore, it is imperative that the communicative skills of children under 3 years of age be assessed in the context of the family system, thus taxing the skills of the EI even further. This is particularly true when the EI realizes that treatment programs for infants and toddlers that attempt to modify caregiver-infant interaction are more effective than those that focus on child behavior alone. Moreover, current legislation requires that planning and intervention involve the child's family. Thus, the EI must acquire the skills necessary to assess communication skills in the context of the family. Hence, early interventionists representing various academic disciplines are working diligently toward developing strategies and assessment tools that afford them the ability to gather samples of socio-communicative behavior that are representative of a child's overall communicative ability. This presents a significant challenge and is reflected in evolving approaches toward the assessment of communicative ability in children under 3 years of age. The intention of this chapter is to alert the EI to a variety of issues relating to the assessment of communication skills. Specific assessment concerns are addressed, as well as a general overview of current assessment practices. Regardless of primary academic discipline, all members of the early intervention team should be aware of the primary role communication skills play in overall development. In addition, all members of the early intervention team should enhance their ability to assess socio-communicative performance in children under 3.

WHY ASSESS INFANTS' AND TODDLERS' COMMUNICATIVE SKILLS?

As was demonstrated in Chapter 1, communicative skills appear to be the developmental domain that consistently separates low-risk from high-risk children, regardless of the reason for risk. Hence, accurate and early follow-up of the communicative status of the populations of children at risk for communicative delay becomes increasingly important. This is particularly true in light of the increasing survival rate for many medically fragile children, as well as for new populations of at-risk children. Why assess the communicative status of infants and toddlers? Five answers emerge.

Early Detection of Communicative Delay

One factor that is consistently tied to the efficacy of early intervention services is age of identification. A specific and detailed discussion of efficacy is presented in later chapters. However, early identification of socio-communicative delay is imperative for maximum improvement in the communicative status of infants and toddlers. Current federal mandate specifies the need for assessment from birth for infants and toddlers with established or at-risk conditions. Several states have expanded this mandate to include those infants and toddlers that are at enhanced risk for developmental delay due to various biologic and/or environmental factors. The move is clearly toward earlier detection of those children who possess or who are at risk of developing delays in their communicative ability. When one recalls the link between communicative skills and school performance and the important role that communicative status plays in overall development, it is easy to understand why significant momentum exists for early detection of communicative delay. In addition, all assessment activity is provided in the context of the family. In recent years, a variety of strategies for observing and measuring the nature of the communicative interchange between caregivers and infants have emerged. These tools and strategies are designed to improve early case finding and detect communicative delay as early as possible. This process leads to an additional reason why early assessment is important.

Decide on Appropriate Intervention

It is impossible to determine whether a child is in need of communicative intervention without accurate assessment. Assessment of communicative skills affords the EI the opportunity to identify whether a delay exists, determine whether intervention is needed, identify child and family strengths, and plot an appropriate course of intervention. The process is set in motion as the EI gains a glimpse into the communicative ability of a child in the family context and makes judgments about the child's need for specific intervention targeting overall socio-communicative performance. Without assessment, the process cannot be set in motion.

Monitor Child and Family Change

Certainly, one important benefit of assessment is the ability to monitor change over time. The issue of serial assessment is discussed in greater detail later in this chapter. However, it should be noted that ongoing assessment is essential if intervention efforts are to be proven effective and if needed changes in the content of intervention are to be made as the child grows and as the family alters its response to the child. Measuring child change has been the method of choice to date in demonstrating the efficacy of early intervention services. Although other measures of efficacy exist (and will be discussed in later chapters) accurate assessment data affords the EI the opportunity to determine the effectiveness of the services a child receives.

Monitor Program Effectiveness

Current early intervention services are delivered throughout the United States in a variety of ways. Some programs provide the bulk of services in the home, others in a center. Significant debate exists relative to the best setting for services. Some services involve the parents from the start and others at a later date. Some strategies are primarily caregiver focused initially and become more child focused over time. What overall program is most effective? Ongoing assessment of communicative skills and abilities affords the EI an opportunity to determine which program of intervention works best. Although this is essentially an efficacy question, it relates to program efficacy. In concert with program efficacy is cost efficacy. Ongoing assessment may afford intervention planners valuable information relative to the most cost-conscious manner in which to deliver services to children under 3 years of age and their families.

Predictive Purposes

One final purpose for assessment of infants and toddlers may lie in the desire to predict long-range outcome for children based on early assessment results. As is demonstrated later in this chapter, accurate prediction is not possible based on early assessment results. Hence, the utilization of assessment data for predictive purposes is tenuous, at best. This is important for the EI to keep in mind because a variety of people (parents, referral sources, and so on) desire some indication of what may lie ahead for a particular child. Although general statements may be made, specific predictions are not possible based on current assessment strategies.

ASSESSMENT OR DIAGNOSIS?

It should be noted throughout this chapter that the use of the word "diagnosis" is avoided. A diagnostic philosophy of assessment has its origins in a medical model of disability. The medical model of disability implies that arriving at a differential diagnosis is essential in plotting a specific course of treatment. Hence, diagnosis dictates treatment, which indicates likely outcome. This is not consistent with an educational model of disability. Although much is known about the contribution of various factors to communicative delay, much remains unknown. Hence, the need to "diagnose" becomes less important. Certainly the need to identify children who possess or who are at risk of developing communicative delay is paramount. However, attaching specific labels to children may be counterproductive and certainly has little to contribute to specific intervention activities. This is particularly true for children who fit the "at-risk" criteria rather than the "established-risk" criteria. Chapter 1 presents a more detailed discussion of at risk versus established risk relative to developmental expectations. In many instances, the EI cannot identify the exact reasons why a particular child displays a pattern of delayed communicative development. There may be a variety of factors—biologic and environmental—contributing to the delay noted. This lack of information, however, does not prevent the child from receiving needed intervention. In other words, the EI does not always need to know why a child has delayed communication performance before initiating intervention. The clinical implications of this are obvious to the experienced EI. There are very few children for whom actual intervention is dramatically different based on diagnosis. Two children may be demonstrating the same level of developmental delay for different reasons. Also, two children may have the same reason for their delay but may be functioning at different developmental levels. In other words, the EI is treating the child's communicative delay and not a specific diagnosis.

MODELS OF CAUSATION

The previous discussion is not meant to suggest that knowledge of causation is insignificant to the EI. It is to suggest that knowledge of causation (why a child is communicatively delayed) should fit into an overall philosophy of viewing etiologically significant factors. One potential manner in which the EI may choose to view etiologically significant factors and how this knowledge affects intervention suggestions is to view causation from either a current or historical perspective. In other words, the EI is encouraged to search for contributing elements to the noted delay. However, a point may be reached at which further inquiry is not of significant benefit to the overall intervention process. Several examples may help to explain the current versus historical model of etiologic factors.

Historical Model

In some instances, the primary reason a child exhibits a delay in communication development is because of events that took place in the past, events over which the EI has no control. These etiologically significant issues are considered to be historical in nature. As such, the exact identification of these factors is not paramount in determining an effective course of intervention. Intervention planning is largely based on the child's present level of function and not the specific disability. Take, for example, the child with Down syndrome. The condition stems from an event that took place in the past. The EI cannot eliminate the presence of Down syndrome. Communication intervention is based on the child's current level of functioning within the family context and not on the child having a specific and identifiable condition. In many instances, the primary reason for disability is rooted in historical events, either prenatal, perinatal, or postnatal in nature. In some instances, these historical events are known; in others they remain unknown. The EI is encouraged to identify significant factors from a historical perspective when possible. But in those instances in which it is not possible to distinguish significant etiologic factors, effort should be directed toward intervention planning and not toward trying to find a reason why.

A corollary issue relative to historical factors relates to what the EI communicates to caregivers. Caregivers want to know why their child is displaying delayed communication development. In some instances, it is possible to identify important factors. In other instances, it is not. It should be communicated to caregivers that the reasons why may never be known and that they should not assume that the delay is their fault. Communication of this nature between caregivers and the EI is of high priority. Recall from the previous chapter that one concern expressed by parents is that there is a lack of effective communication between them and the EI. Open, honest, and direct communication about etiologic factors for an individual child's disability should be fostered. If, over time, the EI is convinced that the caregivers have contributed to the delay noted, this should be carefully communicated to caregivers as they request this feedback.

Current Model

In contrast to the historical model of causation is the current model. In the current model of causation, it is imperative that the EI identify contributing factors to the delay in communication. In fact, identification of current etiologic factors may in large measure direct initial intervention suggestions and recommendations. For example, if a child's communication delay appears to be related to active middle ear infection, then it is imperative that the EI make an appropriate referral for management of the middle ear pathology. In a similar manner, the child that exhibits any one of a number of current and correctable factors that contribute to the delay noted should be referred first for appropriate management. These referrals may even take place prior to the initiation of communication-based intervention, depending on which specific factors apply. In other words, identification of current contributing factors may, at least in part, dictate initial intervention suggestions. The EI is encouraged to remain alert for new developments in the child and/or family that may contribute to a present communication delay. The astute EI realizes that very little remains static when working with children under 3 years of age. So it is important that vigilance be maintained relative to ongoing etiologic issues.

One final comment about models of causation is needed. It is possible that a combination of historical and mixed elements is present in the same child. For example, what about the child with Down syndrome who has current middle ear pathology? Or consider the 15-month-old child with cleft palate who needs additional surgical repair but who would benefit from communication intervention at present? The models identified are not meant to force the EI into a rigid manner of viewing significant etiologic factors. Rather, the models are suggested as a manner in which the EI can place causation in a proper perspective while maintaining a comprehensive picture of a child's early intervention needs.

ASSESSMENT DEFINED

At the outset of this chapter, a definition of assessment was provided. The discussion that follows is directed toward expanding on that definition and making appropriate applications for the EI interested in accurate assessment of communicative performance for children under 3. For the purposes of the following discussion, assessment is defined as "any activity, either formal (through the use of norm-referenced, standardized criteria), or informal (through the use of developmental profiles or checklists) that is designed to elicit accurate and reliable samples of infant-toddler behavior upon which inferences relative to developmental skill status may be made" (Rossetti, 1990a, p. 92). Three key parts of the preceding definition should be stressed. Each of these is discussed in detail in the information that follows.

Any Activity

Assessment is any activity that gathers information about a child's communicative behaviors. A variety of sources of information (activities) are available as part of the assessment process. No one source of information can be considered more important than another. In essence, the EI is encouraged to be alert to information relative to communicative status that may emanate from one of several sources. Several potential sources of information are discussed here.

Parental Data

Certainly the caregiver is one highly valuable source of information regarding communicative status. Careful and detailed information obtained during a caregiver interview is a significant component of effective communication assessment. Parents have consistently shown themselves to be a valuable source of information about their child's communicative behaviors. Although parents may not have a strong ability to interpret their children's communicative behavior, the information provided by parents can assist the examiner in making judgments concerning the child's communication status. Various researchers have demonstrated that parental descriptions of children's behaviors are generally accurate, although their interpretation of behaviors may lack validity (Coplan, 1982; McCormick, Shapiro, & Starfield, 1982). EIs should pay careful attention to descriptive information provided by parents. One helpful tool in conducting a communication-based interview is provided by Rossetti (1990a). This guide represents a directed parent interview that focuses specifically on communication behaviors as part of an overall comprehensive assessment of communicative status. Other tools of this nature are available. The exact tool used is not important. What is important is that the EI learn to listen to and give considerable value to data provided by parents. More recently, the American Academy of Pediatrics has advised member physicians that they should pay particular attention to caregiver concerns about their child's development, suggesting that caregiver concerns are as accurate as formal developmental screening.

Medical Records Report

Medical information can be a valuable source for the EI interested in assessing communicative skills. In part, the child's pertinent medical background becomes the lens through which observed behaviors are interpreted. When possible, a careful parental interview focusing on medical factors and their contribution to communication status should be conducted. In many instances, depending on the setting in which the EI is employed, the child's hospital discharge summary is available. The EI is encouraged to become familiar with the entire range of medical concerns, as well as how these concerns affect the development of effective communication skills. In addition, it is advised that the EI remain as current as possible regarding new and expanding populations of at-risk and established-risk children.

Other EI Reports

Current early intervention services for a given child are most likely delivered within the context of the early intervention team. Hence, the EI concerned with assessing communication skills should be alert to information obtained from other team members. As all EI personnel are becoming better acquainted with the importance of measuring communication status, individual disciplines are directing increased attention toward enhancing observational skills. In many instances, the most valuable samples of behavior are obtained by spontaneous observation. The entire early intervention team should be alert to behaviors that may assist in monitoring overall developmental status and communication status in particular. This is one of the main benefits to a team approach in early intervention and assessment services.

Test Results

Formal test results certainly constitute an indispensable source of information when assessing communication skills. No matter what setting in which the EI is employed, test instruments are used. In some settings, specific instruments may be mandated by state or local service provider guidelines.

Whether through the course of the EI's professional preparation or from other sources, many EIs have assumed that assessment primarily means administering an assessment instrument (test). The experienced EI soon realizes that infant-toddler assessment may be anything but test administration. A test, no matter how complicated to administer or score, is simply a system designed to collect samples of behavior. Although available tests use a variety of systems to assemble and analyze the samples of behavior collected, a test simply is a means of structuring observations and reporting results. As such, there are significant limitations in all available tests.

A critical principle to keep in mind is that the key to constructive communication assessment is not the test used, but rather the proficiency of the assessor. In other words, no test will make a marginally skilled assessor more effective. In fact, the opposite is true. Competent assessors can induce a marginally effective assessment instrument to work for them. The key to assessment, therefore, is not the test chosen, but the competence of the assessor. There are at least three skills critical to effective assessment, and each rests with the assessor. The assessor must become an effective elicitor, observer, and interpreter of the samples of child behavior obtained. In many instances, valuable sources of behavior are ignored by the assessor because they do not fit the protocol afforded by a particular assessment instrument. That is not meant to minimize the importance of tests. It is, however, meant to sensitize the EI to the reality that skill in test administration does not necessarily make one an effective assessor of communication skills. One could argue that the more test dependent the assessor, the less competent. This is particularly true for those who become test dependent.

No shortage of assessment instruments designed for use with children under 3 years exists. The following discussion is not intended to focus attention toward any specific assessment tool. Rather, it is directed toward assisting the EI in forming an overall philosophy of test administration and the appropriateness of various assessment strategies.

NORM-REFERENCED VERSUS CRITERION-REFERENCED TESTS

It does not take long before the EI interested in assessing communicative skills of children under 3 realizes that one of the first choices that must be made in test selection is whether a norm-referenced or criterion-referenced instrument is best. Although there is disagreement among EIs about the merits of one type of test over another, there is a growing conviction among those assessing children less than 3 years of age that norm-referenced tests are inappropriate. The discussion that follows provides the EI with a general philosophy that should guide test selection and that delineates some of the reasons why a movement away from norm-referenced tests for children under 3 is taking place.

Limitations of Norm-Referenced Tests

A norm-referenced test is one that affords the assessor the opportunity to discriminate among the performance of a group of people and thus interpret how an individual's performance compares with that of the group. In essence, a norm-referenced test (NRT) allows the assessor to view an individual's performance with reference to group performance on similar tasks. Although the method of data collection for NRTs may vary, for the most part direct elicitation of desired behaviors by an examiner is used. The outcome of NRTs may be reflected in a variety of ways, including developmental ages, developmental quotients, perceptual quotients, age level scores, mental age or IQ scores, general scale indexes, or overall profiles of global performance (Rossetti, 1990a). For children under 3 years, the use of NRTs has several significant limitations.

Scoring Criteria Narrowly Defined

The nature of norm-referenced instruments requires that the EI keep two important factors in mind. First, the principles of normalization and standardization stipulate that all test items must be administered in a narrowly prescribed fashion. In other words, the test dictates in large measure how the test item must be administered. Second, the manner in which a child responds to test elements must likewise fit a relatively narrow pattern of response. Corollary behaviors that demonstrate comparable performance may not be universally considered in arriving at an overall score for NRTs. Violation of either of these principles places in jeopardy the normalization and standardization of the test for an individual child.

In looking more closely at this principle, one can see the limitations inherent in narrowly prescribing how an item must be administered and scored. For example, most tests employed for children under 3 have items included that are designed to monitor how adequately a child is able to visually track an object. The examiner is generally instructed to place an object (usually a red ball or other red object) within the child's field of vision. The examiner is then instructed to move the object laterally and then up and down. The child is assumed to have a passing score on that particular item if the youngster suitably follows the object (according to the definition provided by the test about what represents appropriate tracking). If the child does not appropriately track the object, the item must be marked as failed. What happens if the child does not track the object but visually attends to someone as they walk across the room? Can that behavior be substituted for the performance required on the test? Generally the answer is no. Conflicts of this nature become common when test administration requires a narrow definition of acceptable behaviors. This is particularly true for children under 3 years. In many instances, the best samples of behavior are not obtained as part of test administration, but spontaneously. It is dichotomies of this nature that are causing many EIs to lean toward using norm-referenced tests, but generally not in the manner in which they were originally intended. In other words, EIs that are using norm-referenced tests are not using or scoring them in the manner intended. Hence, if EIs are not using norm-referenced tests in their intended manner, why use them at all?

Lack of Predictive Ability

Theoretically, one of the main attractions of norm-referenced tests should be the ability to make long-range predictions about a child's developmental performance. In reality this is not possible. For normally developing populations of children, the correlation between norm-referenced developmental test scores and later performance does not approach significance until approximately 3 years of age. In other words, it is not until approximately 3 years of age that test scores have any predictive significance for normally developing children.

The application to populations of infants and toddlers with special needs is readily apparent. The predictive ability of norm-referenced tests is quite low for this group of children. Hence, the value of norm-referenced tests for predictive purposes is questionable at best. A general principle that the EI should remember is that the younger the child, the less predictive norm-referenced test scores will be. Time, spontaneous recovery of function, and maturation are in the child's favor. The EI who attempts to make long-range predictions based on norm-referenced test results for children under 3 years will generally find those predictions to be wrong. This becomes a significant issue because parents and others are seeking information about long-range expectations. Although more is known about long-range expectations for children with established risk (see Chapter 1), the EI is much less able to make long-range statements about children who are at risk based on a single test administration. The information provided to parents based on test administration, if intended to be predictive in nature, can at best be misleading and at worst be completely inaccurate. So the EI is cautioned about using norm-referenced test results in providing parents with long-range statements about a child's performance.

Scoring Difficulties

Three issues should be discussed regarding scoring difficulties when using norm-referenced tests. These relate to item validity, overall scoring, and interpretation of results. A review of existing communication-based assessment instruments reveals that many tests use identical behaviors as part of test administration. Little review of the validity of the behaviors contained in existing tests is available. Recall the example of the eye tracking task mentioned previously. How valid is eye tracking relative to the intent of the test being administered? Many communication-based assessment instruments attempt to measure the average number of words contained in a child's utterances (mean length of utterance, or MLU). How valid a measure of overall communication status is MLU? Perhaps a more valid measure would be the number of communicative attempts a child makes in a given period of time. The point is that the answers to these questions and the overall issue of item validity are currently unavailable. These questions certainly demand more systematic research. At any rate, items contained in current norm-referenced assessment instruments are in need of review.

A second issue relative to scoring NRTs is how overall scores are computed. In general, all items contained on norm-referenced instruments count equally in computing a child's overall score. Items are not weighted. Once an overall score is obtained, it is analyzed in accordance with the instrument's norms. Various interpretations are likely. If item validity is a concern, then perhaps some items are more representative of the test's intent and, therefore, should be viewed as more prominent when scoring. Overall scores appraised in accordance with normalization procedures are of limited benefit when one is attempting to identify specific areas of communication functioning that may or may not reflect delayed performance.

A final subject that must be addressed on norm-referenced test scoring relates to how the results are used in structuring intervention activities. For the most part, norm-referenced test results are of limited value in identifying areas of strength and weakness. One goal for the EI should be a seamless transition between assessment and intervention. Global scores examined in concert with normalization guidelines do not promote such a transition. In many instances, the EI must backtrack and identify a starting point for intervention based on information gained from sources other than norm-referenced test results. NRT results are minimally helpful to the EI for structuring specific communication-based intervention activities.

Criterion-Referenced Tests

The second category of assessment instruments is criterion-referenced tests (CRTs). CRTs are those in which content is defined in terms of some specific performance dimension under investigation. Tests of this nature assess the performance of an individual relative to well-defined performance expectations and indicate mastery or nonmastery of that particular domain. In essence, CRTs provide an overall indication of performance on a well-defined aspect of behavior.

One benefit of CRTs for the assessment of communication skills is that the assessor is allowed to elicit desired behaviors thought to be characteristic of skill mastery in whatever manner best fits a child. So if a child does not name a specific object presented as part of test administration but later names a different object in a spontaneous fashion, the child can be said to have that particular behavior mastered. Administration procedures are not as strict as those for NRTs. The actual administration of the CRT may allow data collection based on behavior directly elicited by the examiner or parental report or from spontaneously occurring behavior. The overall purpose of measures of this nature is to determine an individual's mastery of desired behaviors regardless of the setting or manner in which the behaviors are observed. This is a significant advantage over NRTs.

Perhaps one of the greatest benefits of CRTs over NRTs lies in how the results are used. In essence, CRTs function as a developmental profile or checklist of mastered behaviors. Overall results on CRTs are readily transferred into appropriate intervention suggestions. For CRTs that are comprehensive in nature, behaviors are monitored that are generally not included in NRTs. Accordingly, a relatively seamless progression from test results to intervention recommendations is likely. In addition, as a child demonstrates progress in communication skills, the CRT is more likely to reflect change. NRTs do not immediately reflect change unless a sufficient number of items exhibit improvement, thus supporting an adjustment in scoring procedures and conclusions. It is also much easier to communicate areas of strength and weakness, change evidenced, and new avenues of intervention to caregivers through criterion-referenced assessment results.

The EI interested in accurate appraisal of communication performance in children under 3 years will undoubtedly use available assessment instruments. Employing tests is not the issue. What is of issue is that the EI understand both positive and negative features inherent in categories of assessment instruments, as well as in specific tests under consideration.

Samples of Behavior

One concept that the EI must keep in mind is that during the course of communication assessment all that is available is a limited sample of behaviors. As such, the examiner may elicit a good sample or a bad sample. In other words, a child may or may not display behaviors that are representative of overall communication competence. This understanding, alone, lends an additional reason why assessment results cannot be viewed in a predictive manner. A variety of factors may be present in the child, the setting, the family, and/or the assessment procedures employed that reduce the accuracy of a given sample of communication behaviors elicited in a session.

The following analogy illustrates this concept. Suppose that one individual wishes to learn what the interior of another's home looks like and then describe the home's interior to a group of people. The person investigating the interior of the home has several methods available. The individual might choose to use video recording equipment, a sketch pad, a still camera, or simply rely on memory recall of the home. The task appears relatively simple. The description can be assumed to be accurate and reliable regardless of the methods used. The audience receiving the description would have a much better understanding of the interior of the home under study with any method. However, what would the accuracy of the description of the home be if the person involved in the investigation were permitted to look into only one room? The audience's familiarity with one room would be sound. But the audience's knowledge of the rest of the home would be quite limited. Why would this be the case? Simply because only a limited glimpse into the home was allowed.

This same principle holds true for infant-toddler assessment. The EI has access to a limited sample of behaviors. So the ability to describe the sample obtained is adequate, but the ability to make statements about the child's entire communicative competence would be suspect, at best. One principle to keep in mind following assessment is that one may have obtained a good sample of behaviors or a bad sample of behaviors but certainly not a predictive or exhaustive sample of the child's communicative skills. The EI is encouraged to not be placed into a context in which broad statements about a child's communicative competence and future potential are expected based on a glimpse into a limited sample of behaviors (one room only).

This principle gives rise to a discussion of the value of ongoing, or serial, assessment. Detailed information on the nature of serial assessment, the benefits of such ongoing assessment, and specific issues such as when to start and assessment intervals are presented later in this chapter. The EI is encouraged to continually recall that only limited information is available relative to a child's communicative competence based on a single sample of behaviors.

Inferences

The final aspect of the definition of assessment provided earlier lies in the understanding that the EI is not a diagnostician but rather an inference maker. Previous discussion centered on the question of assessment versus diagnosis. The point was stressed that the EI is not a diagnostician. What then is the assessor?

Although varying terms may be used, one simple manner in which to understand the role the EI plays in assessment is that of inference maker. As an inference maker, the EI is simply inferring whether a sample of behaviors obtained during an assessment reflects age-appropriate expectations. If the sample reflects age-appropriate performance, no further recommendations may be necessary, with the EI inferring that the child is developing normally; the only additional recommendation might include future retesting. However, if the sample of behaviors obtained during the assessment leads the EI to infer that the child is not displaying age-appropriate performance, a whole range of potential recommendations is possible. The content of the recommendations depends in large measure on the child, the family, and specific aspects of the child's communicative delay, including contributing factors to the delay noted. This view of assessment frees the EI from being forced into a diagnostic/predictive mode. It affords the EI the opportunity to structure intervention based on the current level of performance (strengths and weaknesses). Additionally, it allows the assessor the freedom to communicate to caregivers that no one can make long-term predictions based on limited samples of behavior. The EI can then reinforce the need for ongoing (serial) assessment.

The key concept to keep in mind in any discussion of assessment is that the test used is not the most important issue. In a comprehensive view of assessment, test data is only one source of information. Information from all sources should be counted as equally valuable in gaining insight into a child's communication competence.

GENERAL ASSESSMENT PRINICPLES

The information in the following sections is designed to familiarize the EI with a variety of general assessment considerations. One basic principle to bear in mind is that no guaranteed (cookbook) strategy for assessment exists. As has been stressed previously, the key to effective assessment is the assessor and not the instrument used. In fact, in a relatively short time, people with minimal exposure to issues related to early intervention could be trained to administer most available assessment instruments. What sets the EI apart as an effective assessor of communication skills is not the ability to administer tests, but rather the clinical skills necessary to interpret information gained (regardless of the source of the information) and use that information in structuring an effective program of remediation. Each topic discussed in the sections that follow is designed to enhance the EI's understanding of issues important for a thorough assessment of communication skills for children birth through 3 years of age.

Developmental Log

Information gained from caregivers, over time, can be of significant value to the assessor. Hence, the EI is encouraged to facilitate and encourage caregivers to keep and use a developmental log. The benefits of a log of developmental change are obvious. In contrast to the limited sample of behaviors obtained during formal assessment, a developmental log affords the assessor an opportunity to observe, through the parent's eyes, ongoing change in the child. This provides the assessor more than a look into a "single room" of the child's complete communicative ability. Knowledge obtained through a maturational log of skill mastery can assist the EI in the selection of assessment instruments, in the identification of emerging communication skills, and in the adjustment of the child's intervention program. An additional benefit of a log lies in the ability to note child change that would not be noted on formal assessment instruments. In many instances, change is subtle in nature. It is unlikely that it will be noted as part of assessment but quite likely that a caregiver will notice and report it on the log.

The process of keeping a developmental log and the instruction provided to parents are relatively simple. In essence, the caregivers are asked to note in the log each time they observe the child doing something that appears to be new. Parents are asked to record the date and briefly explain the fresh behavior observed. A detailed description is not necessary, although many parents will enjoy keeping the log and provide rich descriptive data regarding the child's development and change. An additional benefit of a log is that it requires the parents to be more than passive observers of their child's progress. Through the process of describing observed changes and with the knowledge that the EI will review their log entries, the parent is more readily invested in the overall intervention process. As such, the log has obvious as well as hidden benefits for the EI, the child, and the caregivers.

Serial Assessment

The rationale for serial assessment is similar to that of the developmental log. Serial assessment affords the EI an ongoing glimpse into the child's behavioral change. Serial assessment involves conducting regular assessments over regular periods of time. The need for serial assessment and the benefits of regular assessment are described by McCarthy (1980) and Murphy, Nichter, and Liden (1982). These are presented in modified form:

1. In a testing situation, the examiner is able to elicit only a limited sample of the child's behavior, at best. If the examiner cannot feel reasonably confident about the sample elicited, it should not be quantified or labeled but simply described.

2. The younger the child, the less reliable predictions will be across dimensions measured.

3. Time, spontaneous recovery of function, and maturation are on the side of the young child and may make liars out of the best assessment tools.

4. Serial assessment provides the only means of measuring developmental patterns and rates of development and change.

5. Serial assessment assists the EI in making decisions about intervention.

6. Serial assessment assists the EI in making decisions about the progress of interventions.

7. Serial assessment is the only means of detecting and monitoring new problems as a child matures.

Two questions arise in any discussion of serial assessment. First, when should assessment of communication skills begin? And second, how frequently should the child be assessed?

In determining when assessment should begin, it should be kept in mind that much is known about risk factors for communication delay. Further, a child does not become communicatively delayed when, at approximately 1 year, the child is not using his or her first word. A variety of processes must be in place before the child is able to use its first meaningful word. These two issues viewed in combination lead the EI to conclude that communication assessment should begin as soon in the child's life as possible. Precursors to the use of meaningful words include interaction, attachment, play, pragmatics, and gesture. These can be monitored from the earliest weeks of a child's life. Thus, it is entirely possible to detect delayed/disordered communication or, at least, those children at enhanced risk of developing delayed communication skills before the emergence of the first word. Monitoring of the development of communication skills for at-risk infants should begin as early as possible.

The second question relates to the frequency of assessments. No rigid rule exists. However, if the EI adopts the view that each assessment represents a limited glimpse into the child's communicative ability, then the greater the frequency, the better. Many EIs are adopting an assessment schedule that sets three assessments during the first year as a goal. This becomes increasingly important as communication with caregivers becomes a concern. For the majority of children under 3 years (75% to 85%) (Rossetti, 1990a), no definitive (established) risk factors will be present. Hence, providing caregivers with concrete information is difficult. However, if the EI is able to view a child's communicative status several times during the first year and if the parents keep a developmental log, then a more expansive view of communication skills emerges. The EI must demonstrate caution in what is communicated to caregivers following a single assessment of communication skills. A diagnostic approach is discouraged. Rather, a prescriptive model of viewing assessment results and communicating with caregivers is suggested. This process translates into a very simple assessment suggestion relating to what is communicated to caregivers. It is suggested that the EI demonstrate extreme caution in suggesting that a child is anything, based on a single sample of behaviors. Given the limitations of one sample of behaviors, the EI will more than often be wrong if long-term statements about communicative performance are provided to parents. What can the EI communicate to parents if the sample obtained, in combination with the child's history, indicates increased potential for delay? It is suggested that the parents be reminded that the statements being made by the EI represent one glimpse into the child's communicative ability. Caregivers can be reminded that the single sample obtained is not predictive, although it may represent less than adequate (age appropriate) performance. A recommendation for intervention may be made; however, long-range predictions are tenuous at best.

Monitoring Patterns of Change

Perhaps the greatest benefit of serial assessment is that it affords the EI the opportunity to observe and monitor patterns of developmental change over time. If only a single assessment result is available to the EI, all that is known is whether the child diverges from age expectations. Divergence may be expressed in a variety of ways, depending on the manner in which the test used measures and describes behaviors noted as part of test administration. However, all that is available, based on a single test administration, is the knowledge of how far a child may be from age expectations. Serial assessment allows the EI to describe more than the gap that exists between test results and age expectations. It furnishes the EI with the prospect of viewing how the gap changes over time. In other words, patterns of change and rate of change become a valuable source of information for the EI. If serial assessment is used, the EI becomes aware that several patterns of change are possible. Each of these patterns will be discussed.

NORMAL-ABNORMAL DEVELOPMENT

One pattern of change that may be detected through serial assessment is characterized by maintenance of the interval between where the child is functioning and where he or she should be functioning. In other words, the degree of delay remains the same over time. This pattern may be referred to as normal-abnormal development. It is a pattern characterized by a normal progression of developmental skill mastery. Skills are learned in a normal sequence but later than expected. This is generally seen in a child who shows progress as a result of intervention, but the rate of progress does not exceed developmentally appropriate transformation. Thus, the child displaying a normal-abnormal pattern of change is not catching up, but neither is the youngster falling behind.

ABNORMAL-ABNORMAL DEVELOPMENT

The second possible paradigm of change is characterized by a widening of the distance between where the child is functioning and where he or she should be functioning. In other words, the child is falling further and further behind, perhaps even while receiving early intervention services. This is generally not a positive sign and may be indicative of the potential for substantial and long-term developmental delay. This pattern may be referred to as abnormal-abnormal development. Children who demonstrate this pattern of change must be monitored closely. The content of their intervention program, the degree of caregiver involvement in the overall services provided, and the professionals involved in intervention must be evaluated on a regular basis in an attempt to reverse the widening of the gulf between age-appropriate skills and the child's level of functioning.

CATCH-UP GROWTH

A third pattern of change that may emerge is known as catch-up growth. Catch-up growth may be defined as an accelerated rate of developmental skill mastery, reducing the gap between where the child is functioning and where he or she should be functioning (Rossetti, 1990a). Inherent in this pattern of change is the demonstration of skill mastery at a rate that exceeds usual maturational growth. The child moves toward age-appropriate performance and at a rate faster than normal skill progression. This is generally viewed as a positive prognostic sign. It may reflect one or all of several factors, including the efficacy of the intervention services provided, the degree of caregiver involvement in the overall process, the health of the child, and the elimination of factors that would tend to impede the child's growth and development.

VARYING DEVELOPMENTAL CHANGE

One final model of change that may emerge as a result of serial assessment is reflected in fluctuations in the degree of distance between where the child is functioning and where he or she should be functioning. These fluctuations may be in either direction. That is to say, the gap may widen for a time and then narrow or remain the same. This pattern of change is often noted in children who continue to experience medical complications and are medically fragile, or those whose environment is also unstable and changing. When healthy, they show progress or at least maintain developmental skill progression. However when ill, they manifest a stretching of the interval between current performance and age-appropriate expectations. Children who manifest this pattern of change should be followed closely so that intervention activities can be maximized during times of health and catch-up growth.

The EI is encouraged to be alert to the patterns of change described. This awareness influences intervention activities, has implications for what is communicated to parents, provides enhanced potential for accurate statements regarding future expectations, and provides for more reliable and accurate understanding of a child's performance at a given time and future needs.

Determination of Infant/Toddler State

The experienced EI soon becomes aware that a variety of factors influence the child's performance on any given day. These factors alter the child's ability to provide samples of behavior upon which reliable inferences about skill status are formulated. Issues such as time of day, setting, who accompanies the child to the assessment, general health, and the child's overall state become important.

Typical Child State

The concept of child state was first discussed by Brazelton (1973). In this discussion, infant/toddler state was described as the child's level of alertness or environmental interaction patterns at a given point in time. This view considers the child's state as the lens through which samples of behavior obtained during assessment are interpreted. For example, if a child is assessed following or during illness, less than representative samples of behavior may be obtained. If state is not considered, the examiner may view behaviors as good examples of the child's behavioral capabilities and make false assumptions about the child's level of function at the time of assessment. For the EI interested in obtaining accurate samples of behavior, determination of child state becomes important. Table 3–1 describes infant states as initially discussed by Brazelton (1973).

A child's state depends on both physiologic and environmental factors. Variables such as hunger, general health at the time of the assessment, overall level of alertness, and where the child is on his or her own wake-sleep cycle certainly influence a child's ability to interact during the administration of an assessment instrument. The EI is

TABLE 3–1   Infant States

State	Characteristics
Sleep State	
Deep sleep	Deep sleep with regular breathing, no activity, no eye movement
Light sleep	Rapid eye movements, random startle movements, sucking movements off and on
Awake State	
Drowsy, semidozing	Eyes opened or closed, eyelids fluttering, movements usually smooth, mild startling noted
Alert	Bright looks, focuses attention on objects, motor activity at minimum
Eyes open	Considerable motor activity, increase in startling, high activity level
Crying	Intense crying, difficult to break through even with novel stimuli

Adapted from *Neonatal Behavior Assessment Scale* (p.1), by T. Brazelton, 1973, Philadelphia: J. B. Lippincott.

encouraged to pay particular attention to the child's state when gathering samples of behavior as part of the assessment process.

At-Risk Child State

The child states summarized in Table 3–1 apply to healthy, normally functioning children. Does the child who is at risk or medically fragile present a different pattern of child states? The answer to that question is yes. The application of the concept of states to at-risk infants is more recent and was first described by Gorski, Davidson, and Brazelton (1979). In the Gorski model, three basic states are described. These states are outlined in the discussion that follows. Although the initial discussion of these states was presented in the context of the child who remains hospitalized, these states can be readily observed in any population of children who display ongoing issues related to health and overall development.

Basically, three child states were described by Gorski's group. Unlike the states described for healthy infants in Table 3–1, the states that apply to sick children are better thought of as stages through which the child passes as the youngster moves from illness to health. No set time line is prescribed as the child passes through these stages. This is in contrast to the states discussed in Table 3–1. For those states it is possible for the skilled assessor to manipulate state behavior based on the child's patterns of response to environmental stimuli. Passage through the states described by Gorski depends in large measure on the overall progress the child makes in recovering from any one of a number of potential physical insults and conditions to which high-risk infants are susceptible. In addition, evidence suggests that environmental overstimulation may prolong the child's time in at least the first of the states described by Gorski et al. (1979).

IN-TURNED STATE

The first state that applies to ill children is referred to as the in-turned, or physiologic, state. This is a time during which normal patterns of interaction between the child and his or her environment are not possible. The child's inability to interact with the environment is caused by two factors. First, the child is ill, perhaps critically so. The child is directing all of his or her limited physiologic energy toward maintaining life support. The child has little ability or energy to direct toward environmental awareness or interaction. Infants in the neonatal intensive care nursery, pediatric intensive care unit, or who have recently recovered from a life-threatening illness often exhibit a time during which they are in-turned. In essence, the child is shutting out the world because of illness. A reasonable analogy would be the adult who is experiencing a severe case of influenza. Such an adult is not at his or her best. Hence, good samples of the adult's skills and abilities cannot be obtained.

There is a second cause that contributes to the child demonstrating an in-turned state. Although not as readily apparent as illness, it is just as powerful. This is related to the degree of sensory stimulation the child receives while critically ill. The following example should serve to illustrate this cause. If a well, healthy infant is placed in a sitting position and a bright light is focused directly on the child's face, the child will show a specific pattern of response. The child will tightly close his or her eyes, attempt to pull away, and react negatively to this noxious stimuli. Once the light is turned off, the child will return to normal. If the light is turned on again, a similar pattern of response will be noted. After three trials, the child will tend to remain in a defensive posture designed to protect it from the aversive stimuli of the light. This is, in essence, an in-turned posture. For children who are hospitalized in intensive care units or for whom ongoing medical considerations are present, the combination of illness and sensory satiation from the nature of the care they receive contributes to their inability to demonstrate patterns of interaction with the environment. Material presented in later chapters describes in greater detail the manner in which the environment may be modified to reduce its contribution to a child remaining in an in-turned state. Suffice it to say at this point that a child's physical condition as well as the care the child receives as a result of its physical condition interact in a powerful manner. The result is that the child can be unable to demonstrate optimal patterns of environmental interaction. Hence, the EI is unable to gather samples of behavior that contribute to an accurate understanding of the child's behavioral competence. The in-turned state is not an optimal time to gain samples of behavior.

COMING OUT

Children come into the world uniquely predisposed to consume it. In fact, one thing that can be counted on in the newborn is the desire to be in contact with the world. Nothing special has to be done. The child is an insatiable consumer of environmental stimuli. During the state previously described, a child's illness and the degree of environmental stimulation generated by the youngster's special needs interfere with the child's predisposition to interact with the world. Once the child gains even minimal capacity to control and maintain physiologic systems, the child will, in most instances, begin to display patterns of behavior that reflect natural attempts to respond to the environment in a more meaningful manner. This stage represents the first active response to the environment and implies a more active response to outside stimuli, both nutritional and social. This is a period when changes in the caregiver environment have an impact on a child's physical well-being and growth. This period is when the child is no longer acutely ill and is able to form attachment to a primary caregiver. It is during this stage that the EI can begin to make preliminary observations on how the child interacts with his or her caregivers and how the youngster interacts with the world in general. This is a time when the child's predisposition to make contact with the environment overpowers the difficult medical complications/conditions to which he or she has been exposed. This is an important time for caregivers, EIs, and the child. Coming out represents a transitional time between acute illness and greater participation with the world. Although movement into this state should be viewed in a positive manner, it should be recalled that children remain medically at risk and may relapse into an in-turned state. Likewise, for the older child who displays ongoing medical complications, passage through the coming-out state may take place more than once.

RECIPROCITY

The final state that should be considered for infants and toddlers who have displayed patterns of illness is known as reciprocity. This state represents an optimal period of environmental opportunity. This is a time when the child is healthy and able to respond to the environment in specific and predictable ways. This state begins when the child is breathing on his or her own and feeding better. It may begin just prior to hospital discharge and continue after the child is in the home setting. Behaviors that may be observed include smiling, vocalizing, and varying patterns of interaction with caregivers. Many of the available assessment instruments assume that the child is in the reciprocal state for proper test administration.

It is recommended that the EI make reference to the state the infant is in during all attempts to gather assessment data. Certainly the child's transition from in-turned to coming out to reciprocity should be monitored. If the child does not display movement through these states, the EI is justified in expressing concern about how well the child is doing overall and with communication skills, in particular. It quickly becomes obvious to the EI that regardless of the age at which an infant or toddler is assessed, particular attention must be paid to the child's state. For the EI to disregard state when interpreting assessment results is to set oneself up for inaccurate impressions and judgments about a child's overall skill status.

One final comment is warranted. It is advisable for the EI to ask parents following any assessment whether an accurate sample of behaviors was obtained. Questions such as, "Is this her best behavior?" or "Is this a good sample of what he can do?" can assist in attaching proper significance to the sample of behaviors obtained as part of assessment.

Correction for Prematurity

One primary factor that places children at enhanced risk for communicative delay is prematurity. Largo, Molinari, Pinto, and Weber (1986) suggest that the EI should expect at least a mild delay in communication development in preterm children. The EI should be particularly alert to the potential for delay in communication skills as a result of prematurity and the array of issues surrounding preterm birth.

The concept of correction for prematurity is not a new one. The principle is simple. If the process of development assessment involves comparing a child on a given day with children of comparable age, then chronological age is paramount in interpreting assessment results. With premature children, the question arises as to which age should be used as a basis for comparison. Should the EI use chronological age or should adjustment be made for the child's degree of prematurity? Thus, two questions arise relative to correction for prematurity. First, should correction for prematurity take place? And second, if correction for prematurity does take place, how long should the EI continue to correct in this manner?

In answering the first question posed relative to correction for prematurity, it is helpful to consider the manner in which newborns interact with the world and whether preterm children of comparable chronological age demonstrate similar patterns of interaction. If healthy newborns are carefully observed, and if measures of their interaction are made and then compared with preterm children of similar age, the healthy newborn generally demonstrates superior skills in interacting with the environment. In other words, if a child born 2 months early is observed at 2 months' chronological age (the point at which it should have been born) and compared to a healthy newborn, the newborn will demonstrate superior engagement with the environment. The conclusion is uncomplicated: Correction for prematurity must be considered.

The second question that must be answered relates to how long correction for prematurity should take place. Some investigators feel that correction should be routine until a child reaches 2 years of age, with others suggesting alternatives. Perhaps one of the most comprehensive investigations on correction for prematurity was conducted by Siegel (1983). In this investigation, correcting developmental test scores for degree of prematurity was studied in matched groups of full-term and preterm children. The children were administered a series of developmental tests at ages 4, 8, 12, 18, and 24 months of age. At each age of test administration, the uncorrected scores of the preterm children were significantly lower than those of the full-term matched children. However, corrected scores for the preterm children during the first year of life were more highly correlated with test scores at 3 and 5 years of age. The implication is that subtracting the degree of prematurity from chronological age expectations for children less than 1 year of age results in a more accurate predictor of later developmental expectations. Additional review of the Siegel data revealed that from 12 months of age on, uncorrected scores displayed a higher correlation with test performance at 3 and 5 years of age. Hence, correcting for prematurity and using the corrected scores in judging developmental performance appears to be a more accurate manner of viewing assessment results, particularly for children under 12 months of age. In the Siegel study, both corrected and uncorrected scores had essentially the same predictive ability relative to performance at 3 and 5 years of age. The author concludes the study by stating that "the use of correction for degree of prematurity may be appropriate in the early months, but after one year of age, there were no significant differences between the predictive ability of the corrected and uncorrected scores" (p. 1187).

Although the ability to predict later performance based on test scores obtained for children under 3 years is not convincing, correction for prematurity until the child reaches 12 to 15 months of age is recommended (Palisano, Short, & Nelson, 1985). It should be noted that these investigations were conducted prior to the current increase in survival for children at younger gestational age. In essence, children are surviving at younger gestational ages. So should correction for prematurity continue longer than 1 year for children at or below 26 weeks' gestational age? Research of this nature is currently under way. However, in the presence of increasing survival for children 23 to 26 weeks' gestation, it seems warranted to correct for prematurity until at least 18 to 20 months of age.

Settings for Assessment

For decades, the primary model of service delivery for children with special needs was for the child to receive needed services in the context of the school, hospital, or clinic. This model is referred to as center-based service delivery. With the advent of early intervention services, the evolution of legislation dealing with services to children under 3 years, and the realization of the importance of family involvement in the process, a model of service delivery that is primarily home based has unfolded.

Home-Based Assessment

An important premise on which later information relative to intervention suggestions will be based is that children learn to communicate through natural interactions with their environment and not in a laboratory. So it makes sense that a naturalistic setting for assessment of communication skills affords the EI a valuable glimpse into the child's communicative competence. The most naturalistic environment in which the EI can assess communication skills is in the home. Although a substantial amount of service is still delivered from a center-based perspective, home-based intervention services, particularly for younger children, are gaining acceptance. There are benefits as well as liabilities inherent in home-based communication assessment. The discussion that follows is designed to alert the EI to these issues.

Filler (1983) lists several benefits intrinsic to home-based services:

1. Parents feel comfortable in their own home and therefore act more naturally.

2. Similarly, children are more likely to perform better in their own home. It affords a more naturalistic setting in which to elicit behaviors on which developmental adequacy may be judged.

3. The child's health is better protected. This is of particular importance for children who are medically fragile.

4. Parent and child routines are minimally interrupted. As a result, a more accurate sample of parent-child interaction may be obtained.

5. There is a greater likelihood of gaining helpful insights because other family members are present.

Although a specific database examining the efficacy of home-based assessment services does not exist, there is information relative to the effectiveness of home-based intervention services available. In a report to the chairman of the Subcommittee on Labor, Health and Human Services, Education, and Related Agencies, Committee on Appropriations, U.S. Senate (1990), a variety of positive outcomes of home-based services were presented. Evaluations of early intervention programs using home visiting demonstrated that home-based programs can improve both the short- and long-term health and well-being of families and children. In this report, home visiting was defined as a strategy that delivers health, social support, or educational services directly to individuals in their homes. Programs engaged in home-based services use home visitors of various disciplines and skills to accomplish various goals and provide various services. The report further specifies that, with the evolution of aggressive legislation designed for children and their families, home visiting should increase as a service delivery option. The report concludes by indicating that the full effects of home visiting for the provision of early intervention services can become more impressive as parents use what they have been taught and children grow and develop further. Such contact during the child's early years results in improved family functioning, better school performance, and better educational outcomes long term.

As is true with any strategy for service delivery, there are several liabilities that accompany home-based assessment. Although these cautions do not outweigh the benefits of home-based assessment, they should be kept in mind by the EI. First, the EI must be alert to the potential for a wide range of responses while in the home setting. A basic premise to keep in mind is that over time the EI may experience practically anything while engaged in home visits. This is both a benefit and liability. In many urban settings, the EI must follow strict rules for personal safety and security. In addition, parents may feel so comfortable that they all but ignore the EI. They may assume that the "professional" has arrived to assess the child, not fully understanding that assessment involves gaining insight into the pattern of interaction that exists between the parent and the child—and that they are an integral part of the process. Although uninvolved parents are discouraging to the EI, those who show patterns of disinterest provide the EI with valuable insight into the communicative environment in which the child functions. An additional caution intrinsic to the home setting is the overall nature of the home environment. The home setting may be maximally distracting to the assessment process. Hence, less than optimal samples of communicative behavior may be obtained. Attempting to assess a child while other children are running around, while the TV is on, or while the parent has his or her attention directed elsewhere is counterproductive to effective assessment. The EI providing home-based assessment or intervention services must always remember that those services are being delivered on someone else's "turf" and that there are cautions inherent in functioning in a home setting.

One final comment relative to home-based services is needed. It is not possible, in most instances, for a large number of EI personnel to visit an individual child's home. Hence, the need for team functioning in a transdisciplinary format is apparent. The concept of transdisciplinary functioning is developed later in this chapter.

Center-Based Assessment

The second environment in which infant-toddler communication assessment activity might be provided is in a center-based delivery system. A center-based service delivery system implies that the child is taken to an intervention setting for appropriate assessment services. There are a variety of settings for center-based activity. These include schools, hospitals, community-based clinics, child development centers, university centers, private practice settings, and rehabilitation facilities. The exact makeup of the personnel involved in center-based settings varies. As with home-based services, both benefits and liabilities exist. Filler (1983) lists several benefits of center-based assessment services. These are listed in modified form:

1. Parents and children have greater access to staff and more services. One of the strengths of the center-based model is that additional professional expertise is readily available. Depending on the general model of service delivery employed, the child may be seen by the entire EI team or at least by one or two assessors.

2. Parents are afforded the opportunity to interact with other parents. The benefits of this interaction should not be underestimated. It is important that parents of infants and toddlers who are disabled realize that they are not alone in their experiences. It is very supporting for parents to have another set of parents with whom they might express frustrations and common experiences.

3. If any specialized services are needed, these are more readily available to the child in a center-based setting.

The liabilities of a center-based system relate to the nature of the environment in which services are delivered. For many children, especially if they are younger and medically fragile, transportation to the center involves tremendous effort on the part of the parent. Child care may be needed, transportation may be a problem, adaptive environments may not be fully available, weather may interfere with regular attendance, and the extra time involved in keeping appointments may stress the family even more. Early intervention providers who are center based are continually working to enhance the ability of parents to be able to keep scheduled appointments with a minimum of effort. As is discussed in greater detail in later chapters, a growing number of early intervention programs use a combination of home- and center-based services. This combined approach appears to be gaining acceptance.

TEAM MODELS OF ASSESSMENT

Any discussion of infant-toddler assessment must include a discussion of the various models of service delivery. Current models of early intervention service delivery reflect an evolution process that is still taking place. Each existing model of team functioning reflects both historical and technological advances and educational thought relative to people with special needs. It is not within the scope of the present chapter to discuss, in detail, this evolution. However, brief reference to team models and the strengths and weaknesses of each is appropriate. Greater time will be directed to a discussion of the most current model of service delivery used for children under 3 years of age and their families. This model, known as the transdisciplinary model, is applied to the assessment of infants' and toddlers' communication skills in the context of assessment paradigms. Basically, there are three models of team functioning. These are the multidisciplinary, interdisciplinary, and transdisciplinary approaches. For a more complete discussion of the evolution of each model, see Foley (1990).

The *multidisciplinary approach* represents a parallel model of service delivery. In this model, professionals tend to work next to each other but with minimal exchange of information or interaction among disciplines. The child may be assessed individually by several early intervention professionals. The professionals involved may be determined by the team leader or someone else in charge of planning for an individual child. This is most generally the physician if the services are hospital based or the psychologist if services are school based. Assessment tends to be discipline specific and conducted separately. Generally, separate reports are generated and submitted to the team leader, who synthesizes the information and organizes a treatment program. The provided intervention likewise tends to be very discipline driven, with little if any overlap between disciplines. Treatment may or may not reflect group consensus. Generally, the family is not viewed as an integral part of the intervention provided. All activities are highly child centered, with little emphasis on involving the family in planning, intervention, or measuring outcomes. In the context of current early intervention mandates and activities, it is easy to see why this model does not fit.

The *interdisciplinary approach* reflects a more cooperative and systematic effort among disciplines. This model moves beyond the notion of working next to one another and moves toward an ideal of cohesion among group members (Hutt, Menninger, & O'Keefe, 1947). This approach continues to stress discipline-specific assessment in a standard fashion. Each professional functions in his or her discipline-specific prescribed role. However, following the assessment phase of intervention, the group meets to exchange information, discuss etiology, agree on diagnosis, and prescribe treatment recommendations in a manner that reflects some degree of group consensus. Foley (1990) describes this approach as "each clinician coming to the meeting with a puzzle piece gleaned from individual assessment, and efforts are made to assemble a configuration that makes sense out of the patient's problem" (p. 273).

A holistic view of health care, an explosion of research in infant development, and the early intervention movement have worked together over the past 10 years to give rise to the *transdisciplinary approach* to team functioning. The transdisciplinary approach has been described as a team model in which a conscious effort to pool and exchange information, skills, and knowledge takes place among disciplines. It is characterized by a crossing and recrossing of traditional disciplinary boundaries by various team members. In the model, as applied to developmental assessment, the child is assessed simultaneously by multiple professionals (arena assessment) representing varying disciplines. The family becomes an integral part of the assessment process. The assessment is more longitudinal, naturalistic, process oriented, and family centered than traditional discipline-specific assessments (Foley, 1990). A common sample of behavior is elicited from which all the professionals involved derive their inferences—generally done in the context of play. This is followed by a meeting of all involved to formulate an integrated report and a cross-disciplinary intervention program. Following the assessment phase, an EI professional (any of the disciplines that participated in the assessment) serves as primary provider of services in conjunction with family participation in the intervention process. This service delivery model is integrative and characterized by role release, role expansion, and arena evaluation for all professionals. Role expansion is the educational, conceptual, and administrative adjustments that must occur to support transdisciplinary practice. Arena evaluation is the simultaneous assessment of the child by multiple professionals of differing disciplines. Role release is intervention focused and refers to the process of transferring specific skills, strategies, and techniques across disciplines to achieve integrated therapy (Foley, 1990).

A growing number of early intervention programs are providing services in this fashion. It differs markedly from the manner in which the bulk of EI personnel have been trained. However, it represents the future of early intervention and is a model that is highly successful.

Transdisciplinary Play-Based/Arena Assessment

In recent years the value of play as applied to assessment paradigms has gained increased interest and acceptance. Play, as used in the assessment of communication skills, involves a facilitator interacting with a child in a play context while gaining samples of communication skills for the purpose of measurement. The premise is that by eliciting, observing, and describing infants' and young children's play behavior, the EI gains significant insight into a child's developmental level. Knowledge of this nature provides a functional baseline of a child's developmental standing and gives rise to appropriate intervention activities. Play itself can be monitored. In addition, play can be employed as a medium for collecting samples of the child's functional skills in other developmental domains as well. This is a growing trend in infant-toddler assessment and one that merits further study and discussion. Casby (1992) states that observation of infant's play, in particular symbolic play, can be an informative and powerful assessment strategy for those engaged in early intervention activities. Hence, the evolution of an assessment strategy that incorporates the importance of play and the realization of the efficacy of transdisciplinary functioning has resulted. This assessment strategy is referred to as transdisciplinary play-based assessment (TPBA).

Transdisciplinary Play-Based Assessment

Transdisciplinary play-based assessment involves the child in structured and unstructured play situations with, at varying times, a facilitating adult, the parent(s), and another child or children (Linder, 1993). This strategy provides an opportunity for developmental observations of cognitive, social-emotional, communication and language, and sensorimotor developmental domains. The method is designed for children between infancy and 6 years of age. A primary proponent of TPBA is Linder (1993).

A review of existing literature relative to TPBA suggests that the benefits of this approach for children under 3 years of age center on the fact that it is functional, natural, holistic, transdisciplinary, and dynamic. By its very nature, flexibility is built into the process. It allows the sequence and content of the assessment to change based on the specific needs and response patterns of the individual child being assessed. One important key to effective TPBA is communication between professionals involved, including the parents, during the evaluation. The process is dynamic and ongoing and represents an approach to assessment that many EI personnel have not been trained to implement; therefore, reluctance to adopt this strategy can be encountered. This reluctance is stronger in an assessment context in which "test completion" is viewed as the main purpose of developmental assessment. A comparison of TPBA and traditional assessment is presented in Table 3–2.

Linder (1993) discusses three main benefits of TPBA. First, TPBA is better able to identify service needs. Examination of a child's performance in various developmental domains can assist the EI team in determining the type and amount of intervention the child may need. Second, information is obtained about a child's functioning in varying situations (play), perhaps with differing examiners. Hence, the development of appropriate intervention plans is facilitated. This information is used in formulating individualized family service plans (IFSPs) or individualized education plans/programs (IEPs). Information gained through TPBA is likely to be more process oriented, functional, and meaningful as the team attempts to devise effective EI programming. Finally, TPBA can be of benefit in evaluating the progress and effectiveness of intervention activities. In many instances, children demonstrate subtle progress in functional ways. This progress may be elusive and not easily detected through standard assessment procedures and instruments but is noted during play activities. This is a significant advantage of TPBA because many available assessment instruments are insensitive to small changes in a child's performance and mastery of developmental skills. Table 3–3 summarizes additional information related to TPBA.

Arena Assessment

A significant expansion of TPBA is transdisciplinary play-based arena assessment. Arena evaluation is the simultaneous assessment of the child by multiple professionals of differing disciplines. A helpful description is provided by Foley (1990), who states that "rather than each professional looking at the child through his/her own individual window, the team designs a picture window so that a common

TABLE 3-2   Comparison of Traditional versus Play-Based Assessment

Disadvantages of Transdisciplinary Traditional Assessment	Advantages of Transdisciplinary Play-Based Assessment
Unnatural Environment • Generally center based • Focus on test materials • Limited room for spontaneous behavior	Natural Environment • May be center or home based • Informal atmosphere, familiar toys, freedom to explore
Unfamiliar Examiner • Adults are unfamiliar to the child • Rapport must be established • Child is in response mode and usually does not initiate interaction • Communication is restricted, emphasis is on test completion	Rapport with Examiner • One examiner through play elicits child's responses • Examiner does not take the lead, the child does • The examiner imitates, models, suggests, and only rarely requests • Structured tasks saved until later
Biased Tests • Biased against children with sensory deficits, communication delay • Tests are generally domain specific and not global in nature	Flexibility in Testing • Adapts to the child and not the tests being administered • Variation in assessment sequence possible • Flexibility in how examiner interacts with child
Structure of Instruments • Presume an invariable sequence of development • Each item equally weighted in arriving at overall score • Individual items may lack validity/reliability • Do not identify subtle changes over time	Holistic Assessment • All team members observe at same time • More global picture of performance possible • Team discussion of child behaviors very positive • Jargon reduced as entire team has observed the same behaviors
Lack of Process Information • Tests yield numbers not information regarding child's learning style strengths/weaknesses	Process Information • Learning style, temperament, mastery motivation, and process observations possible
Lack of Functional Assessment • Tests generally do not assess functional skills	Helps Plan Intervention • Functional skills better assessed; results in better intervention planning
Inappropriate Tests • Children labeled as "untestable" if difficult to test; different assessment methods/tests needed	Every Child Is Testable • Assessment is based on whatever the child is able to do, not what the test dictates

(continued)

TABLE 3-2 (continued)

Disadvantages of Transdisciplinary Traditional Assessment	Advantages of Transdisciplinary Play-Based Assessment
• Child's age may fall between available test suggestions or utilization	Saves Time • Several examiners observe child simultaneously
Time and Cost of Assessment • Child sees a succession of professionals • Separate reports generated • Several assessment appointments may be needed • Staffing takes time	• Joint report generated Involvement of Parents • Parents observe same behaviors as examiners • Parents are part of process, not passive onlookers • Parents feel part of the team
Lack of Other Information • Temperament • Mastery motivation • Interaction patterns	

sample of behavior can be collected" (p. 277). This concept is in full partnership with TPBA. One driving assumption behind arena evaluation is that discrete assessment by multiple professionals is questionable. Each professional interprets behavior through his or her own disciplinary bias. The potential for seeing several different children as each evaluates the same child is enhanced. One concept that is integral to arena assessment is that of role release. Role release is the process of transferring specific skills, strategies, and techniques across disciplines with the goal of achieving comprehensive and integrated assessment outcomes. Haynes (1983) describes the process of role release as having four component parts. Although these were initially presented in the context of intervention, they are readily adaptable to the process of assessment.

First, a primary facilitator must be chosen. This choice may be based on experience, training, and general goodness of fit with a child, family, and referring problem. Second, the specific content of the assessment that is to be role released should be discussed by the team. Communication between team members is paramount to the success of an arena assessment. Third, formal training between team members should be conducted. This is designed to assist each team member in better understanding the types of behavior each professional might be interested in as part of the assessment process. Finally, ongoing follow-up and consultation between all team members is essential. This guarantees back-and-forth communication

TABLE 3-3   Summary of Transdisciplinary Play-Based Assessment

Who Can Be Assessed?
Children functioning developmentally between infancy and 6 years of age
can be assessed. TPBA may be used for children with no disability, who are
at-risk, or for whom other means of assessment are not appropriate.

Who Can Conduct a TPBA?
The number and variety of professionals involved in TPBA may vary at any
given time. The parents (caregivers) are an important part of the process.
Basically, anyone with general or specific knowledge regarding child
development may participate.

How Are Parents Involved?
Parents are involved throughout the TPBA process. Historical information is
provided by parents, and information may be added during the course of the
assessment. Parents may also be part of the play activities.

Where Is TPBA Conducted?
Any suitable play environment can be used for TPBA. The setting and toys
used should be chosen to facilitate exploration, manipulation, problem-
solving behaviors, communication and language, and emotional expression.

What Does TPBA Involve?
In essence TPBA is both an assessment and intervention procedure. Initial
information gathered from parents is used to preplan a play session. Once
the child is comfortable in the play setting, the parents may gradually
withdraw from the interactions. The process is a five-phase one. Phase 1 is
unstructured facilitation, in phase 2 more formal play is incorporated, phase
3 involves the introduction of a peer, phase 4 includes parental
interaction/play with the child, and the final phase involves an eating activity.

Adapted from *Transdisciplinary Play-Based Assessment: A Functional Approach toward Working with Young Children* (p. 163), by T. Linder, 1993, Baltimore: Paul H.
Brookes.

between the role-releasing and role-receiving members of the team.
Role release does not come easily and may be a source of considerable
apprehension and anxiety among EI professionals. The key to effective arena assessment is role release and the key to effective role
release is trust. Foley (1990) identifies three attributes as being essential for effective role release. These are a feeling of confidence and
positive identity, an ability to share and derive feelings of self-worth
and accomplishment from cooperative effort, and a knowledge that
one's professional identity is derived as much as from what one
knows as from what one does. The critical skill in arena assessment is
not in the administration of tests but in collecting a range of behaviors
and in interpreting behaviors in a manner that affords reliable inferences regarding a child's developmental skill mastery and status. The
overall philosophy inherent in arena assessment is that a range of

professionals is allowed to solicit, observe, and interpret a developmental slice of life. Although specific test instruments may be used, there are few instruments designed specifically for transdisciplinary arena assessment. The key is not the tests used but rather the team's ability to elicit and effectively interpret the samples of behavior obtained. Table 3–4 presents an outline of the outcomes expected as a result of transdisciplinary arena assessment.

SPECIFIC COMMUNICATION ASSESSMENT DOMAINS

Communication skills represent one of the foremost developmental abilities included as part of overall infant-toddler assessment.

TABLE 3–4 Outcome of Transdisciplinary Arena Assessment

Historical and Contextual Information
A descriptive review of the medical and social background of the child and the family is gained.

Qualitative Descriptions of the Child's Function
This information provides data relative to how the child interacts with the world. It is more functional than psychometric in nature.

Quantitative Assessment of Functional Levels
This information relates to psychometric issues relative to measurement of how the child interacts with the world. It answers the "how much" questions.

Identification of Dysfunctional Development
This involves the identification of deficits in any area of development and how these deficits affect other areas of skill mastery.

Developmental Formulation
Causal links between behaviors observed, historical information and the development of the problem are identified.

Diagnosis
A formal diagnosis may or may not be reached. Whatever the outcome, a group decision is the goal.

Integrated Transdisciplinary Report
Discipline-specific information is included (interwoven) into the report. This is no small task and must be worked toward.

Transdisciplinary Intervention Planning
This plan, constructed by the team, serves as a comprehensive blueprint to intervention. It affords the primary interventionist access to all areas of suggested intervention derived from one source.

Adapted from "Portrait of an Arena Evaluation: Assessment in the Transdisciplinary Approach" (p. 185), by G. Foley in *Transdisciplinary Assessment of Infants*, edited by E. Gibbs and D. Teti, 1990, Baltimore: Paul H. Brookes.

Communicative adequacy, highly correlated with later developmental performance, is more than a simple accounting of the number of words understood or spoken by an individual. There are several components of effective communicative performance. The information following is not meant to be an exhaustive discussion of each of these components. Rather, it is meant to alert the EI to the complexity of effective communicative assessment. A list of assessment tools designed to assist the EI in effective evaluation of communication skills for children under 3 years of age is presented in the appendix at the end of the chapter. More comprehensive coverage of communication assessment is provided by Capute and Accardo (1991), Coggins (1991), Linder (1993), Rescorla (1991), Rossetti (1990b), Theadore, Maher, and Prizant (1990), and Sparks (1989).

Assessment of Infant-Caregiver Interaction

It is well established that many infants are not afforded an optimal opportunity to form a stable relationship with a primary caregiver. The child who spends the first weeks of life in an intensive care nursery simply has limited energy to direct toward interacting with its caregivers. In addition, during a child's prolonged periods of hospitalization, caregivers have limited opportunity to provide direct, hands-on care for their baby. Hence, both parents and infants must get to know one another sometime after the child is in the home setting. This may take place many days after the birth of the child. The overall pattern of medically oriented care during hospitalization precludes the child and mother from establishing early and effective interactional patterns.

Sparks, Clark, Oas, and Erickson (1988) note that interaction cues and responses of infants include eye contact, crying, quieting, attention to faces and voices, and body movements. They further point out that infant-caregiver interactions that are in synchrony are thought to have long-term effects on cognitive, social, and linguistic skills. It is precisely behaviors of this nature that form the basis of assessment of maternal-infant interaction. The importance of early mother-infant interactions is further supported by information provided by Jacobsen, Starnes, and Gasser (1988). These authors note that mothers who do not talk frequently to their premature infants generally have children who score lower on developmental scales than children who have received sufficient interaction. This finding has powerful implications for the EI and should be part of any attempt to monitor mother-infant interaction.

Klein and Briggs (1986) have devised a scale designed for use in observing the communicative interactions that take place between mother and infant. The Observation of Communication Interaction (OCI) was developed for use as an informal observation guide to assist EIs in describing interaction strategies used by parents. Its main benefit is that it assists in formulating a qualitative assessment of strengths and weaknesses in caregiver interaction patterns. The results of the OCI may be used for planning individual target goals, intervention strategies, and interaction activities. The OCI is administered during a routine caregiving activity between mother and infant. Problems in mother-infant interaction can be readily identified, with specific intervention strategies targeted. Table 3–5 presents an adapted scoring form based on the OCI.

An additional strategy to monitor mother-infant interaction is provided by Walker and Thompson (1982). The Mother Infant Play Interaction Scale (MIPIS) is designed for use in rating live or taped interactions of mothers and infants 4 to 6 weeks after birth. It is administered during a 5-minute session of unstructured play, generally in the home setting. It was devised to measure strategies that mothers use to elicit social behaviors from their infants and, in turn, describe how infants respond to these initiative attempts by the mother. Table 3–6 summarizes several aspects of interaction that the MIPIS evaluates. Farran, Clark, and Ray (1990) present a more complete discussion of specific interaction assessment instruments. Whatever method is used by the EI, it should be kept in mind that a qualitative description of parent-child interactions is a helpful supplement to understanding the family before an intervention plan is established.

Information of this nature should be viewed as another piece of a larger puzzle in fully understanding a particular child in the context of the family. In some instances, the assessment of parent-child interactions becomes the primary focus of intervention planning. Effective intervention is predicated, in many instances, on building on a family's existing strengths. The assessment of parent-child interaction allows the EI the opportunity to focus not only on areas of weakness but also on positive issues for the child in the context of the family.

Assessment of Infant-Caregiver Attachment

Closely related to the monitoring of maternal-infant interaction is the observation of maternal-infant attachment. The previous chapter

TABLE 3–5 Observation of Communicative Interaction Scoring Sheet

ITEM	RARELY/NEVER	SOMETIMES	OFTEN
1. Caregiver provides appropriate tactile and kinesthetic stimulation (strokes, caresses, pats, cuddles, and rocks baby).			
2. Caregiver displays pleasure while interacting with baby.			
3. Caregiver responds to child's distress.			
4. Caregiver positions self and infant so eye-to-eye contact is possible (facing and 7–12 inches away).			
5. Caregiver smiles contingently at infant.			
6. Caregiver varies prosodic features (higher pitch, talks slower, exaggerated intonation).			
7. Caregiver responds contingently to infant's behavior.			
8. Caregiver encourages conversation.			
9. Caregiver modifies interaction in response to negative cues from infant.			
10. Caregiver uses communication to teach language and concepts.			

Adapted from *Observation of Communication Interaction Scoring Sheet (OCI), Observation of Communicative Interaction: A Model Program to Facilitate Positive Communication Interactions between Caregivers and Their High-Risk Infants*, by D. Klein and M. Briggs, 1986, DHHS Publication No. MCJ 06351-01-0, Washington, DC: U.S. Government Printing Office.

pointed out the tenuous nature of maternal-infant attachment when a child is born early, ill, or with special needs. If caregiver involvement in intervention is important for the efficacy of early intervention ser-

TABLE 3-6　Mother-Infant Play Interaction Scale
Items

- Maternal holding style
- Maternal expression of affect
- Maternal caregiving style
- Predominant infant wakeful response level
- Predominant infant mood and affect
- Maternal visual interaction
- Infant visual interaction
- Style of play—animate versus inanimate interaction
- Maternal vocalization style—general (tone and content)
- Maternal vocalization style—quantity of contingency
- Maternal attempts at smile elicitation
- Kinesthetic quality of interaction
- Synchrony of affect
- Termination of interaction

Adapted from "Mother Infant Play Interaction Scale" (p. 29), by L. Walker and E. Thompson in *Analysis of Current Assessment in the Health Care of Young Children and Childbearing Families*, edited by S. Humenick-Smith, 1982, Norwich, CT: Williams & Wilkins.

vices and if difficult early experiences have the potential to impede the formation of proper maternal-infant attachment, then strategies designed to assist the EI in monitoring maternal-infant attachment are important. As has been previously pointed out, attachment may be defined as a unique relationship between two people that lasts over time (Klaus & Kennell, 1976). A lack of attachment during the early months can translate into later caregiving deficiencies. These can be made worse if the child is ill for a prolonged period of time. A wide range of stressful factors may take place that can profoundly influence a woman's subsequent mothering behavior and, ultimately, her child's developmental performance.

One strategy that has gained acceptance as a method for monitoring maternal-infant attachment is the Strange Situation Procedure (Ainsworth, Blehar, Waters, & Wall, 1978). The Strange Situation Procedure focuses on the infant and an attachment figure (generally the mother). The intent of the procedure is to observe how the infant organizes his or her behavior with the caregiver and an unfamiliar person in an unfamiliar environment across several sessions. These sessions vary in their ability to elicit infant distress. The focus of the procedure is to note patterns of infant behavior during separations and reunions with the caregiver and to the presence of an unfamiliar adult. This procedure is generally used with infants between 10 and 24 months of age. The procedure consists of eight episodes and their content. It is during these episodes that the infant is exposed to a variety of strange situations in which various observations are made. Table 3–7 describes six dimensions that are measured as part of the scale. It is from these dimensions that major patterns of attachment are noted and described.

From these rating scales (Table 3–7), Ainsworth and colleagues (1978) describe three major patterns of attachment. These are pattern A (Avoidant), with two subgroups; pattern B (Secure), with four subgroups; and pattern C (Resistant), with two subgroups. Pattern A infants generally demonstrate avoidance of the caregiver by showing no greeting or delayed greeting on reunions. Additional manifestations of avoidance may include playing with their back to the caregiver, avoiding eye contact, and/or ignoring the caregiver's social bids. Pattern B infants typically greet the caregiver promptly and show some degree of seeking of the caregiver, with low levels of avoidance or resistance noted. Infants who fit this pattern show the ability to use the caregiver as a secure base to explore the environ-

TABLE 3–7   Dimensions of the Strange Situation Procedure

Proximity and contact-seeking behavior: Assesses the vigor and quality with which the infant seeks the proximity of and contact with the caregiver or stranger.

Contact-maintaining behavior: Measures the degree to which the infant strives to maintain contact with the caregiver or stranger once contact has been achieved.

Resistant behavior: Indexes the degree of resistant, angry, fussing, petulant behavior directed toward the caregiver or stranger.

Avoidant behavior: Assesses the degree to which the infant avoids or snubs the caregiver or stranger.

Distance interaction: Rates the amount of positive social interactive bids the baby directs to the caregiver or stranger.

Search behavior during separations: Indexes the amount and intensity of searching for the caregiver that takes place when the child is separated from the caregiver.

Adapted from *Patterns of Attachment: A Psychological Study of the Strange Situation* (p. 210), by M. Ainsworth, M. Blehar, E. Waters, and S. Wall, 1978, Hillsdale, NJ: Lawrence Erlbaum Associates.

ment. If distressed, they tend to soothe quickly. During play they may tend to occasionally check on the location of the caregiver. During stressful situations, these infants derive security from the presence of the attachment figure. Type C babies differ markedly. They are noted for repeated expressions of anger, crying, pouting, whining, and the like. These behaviors may be particularly apparent during reunion situations. Infants who fit this pattern may be hard to soothe or console by either the caregiver or stranger.

The use of the Strange Situation Procedure for populations of at-risk infants has received increasing attention in recent years. There is substantial literature demonstrating the usefulness of the procedure for sick and disabled infants without evidence of cognitive delay. One population of infants for whom the Strange Situation Procedure has been called into question is children with Down syndrome. In general, the procedure is not suggested for infants for whom an intellectual/cognitive delay is suspected. For additional information on the Strange Situation Procedure and additional attachment assessment strategies, see Teti and Nakagawa (1990).

Assessment of Play

Various researchers have demonstrated interest in play behaviors relative to the development of communication skills. Early writings, primarily by Piaget, described ordered stages of play during several periods of the child's life. More recent research has sought to further describe, objectify, and verify the content and developmental order of play development, as well as the relationship between play and communication performance. This interest has more recently been directed toward the nature of symbolic play activities and communication development for young children with developmental disabilities. The application of play assessment for populations of children with special needs assumes that by eliciting, observing, and describing infants' and young children's play behaviors, the EI may be able to gain significant insight into the child's overall development. Hence, knowledge of the infant's and young child's level of play provides a functional baseline of the child's developmental level and may provide additional direction for intervention efforts (Casby, 1992).

The relationship between symbolic play and communication development is well established (Terrell & Schwartz, 1988). Several models for better understanding play behavior have been suggested. One, described by Mindes (1982), is presented in Table 3–8. This

TABLE 3-8 Definitions of Play Categories

Social Play

> ***Solitary play:*** The child plays alone with toys different from those used by other children; the child is centered on self-activity.
>
> ***Parallel play:*** The child plays independently but among other children; the child plays beside rather than with other children.
>
> ***Group play-associative play:*** The child plays with other children; all engage in similar if not identical activity.
>
> ***Cooperative play:*** The child plays in an organized group; there is a sense of belonging and an organization in which the efforts of one child are supplemented by the other children.

Cognitive Play

> ***Functional play:*** Simple muscular activities and repetitive muscular movements with or without objects are used in functional play; the child repeats or initiates actions.
>
> ***Constructive play:*** The child learns the use of play materials and attempts to create something with play materials.
>
> ***Dramatic play:*** The child takes on a role and pretends to be someone else using real or imagined objects.
>
> ***Games with rules:*** The child accepts and adjusts to prearranged rules.

Miscellaneous Play

> ***Unoccupied behaviors:*** The child is not playing in the usual sense but watches activities of momentary interest.
>
> ***Onlooker behavior:*** The child watches others play.
>
> ***Reading:*** The child is being read to by an adult caregiver.

Adapted from "Social and Cognitive Aspects of Play in Young Handicapped Children," by G. Mindes, 1982, *Topics in Early Childhood Special Education, 2*, p. 90.

model views play in three distinct categories, with various subcategories under each main heading. Although not presented in an assessment format, this information can be helpful to the EI in gaining a more complete understanding of the nature of play and of the different functions of play in the developing child. What is currently known about changes in play activity is that children's play behaviors undergo a shift during the first 2 years of life. This shift is characterized by a move from undifferentiated activity toward single objects to behavior that is modified to fit the characteristics of individual objects, to functional play involving interrelationships between objects, and finally to symbolic use of objects. Bond, Creasy, and Abrams (1990) summarize at least three trends that emerge in play during the first 2.5 years of life. These trends, which are thought to reflect early cognitive developmental transitions, are (1) decentration, in which symbolic actions are freed from the child's own body; (2) decontextualization, in which pretend play becomes increasingly independent of environmental support; and (3) integration, leading first to sequentially and then hierarchically organized play.

Two general strategies for assessing child play have emerged. One strategy is predicated on unobtrusive observation of a child's free play. The second strategy (structured elicitation) involves explicit attempts to elicit an optimal level of cognitive performance through modeling and/or verbal instructions (Bond et al., 1990).

Free-play observations vary in the degree to which they employ naturalistic versus more structured settings. In a more naturalistic approach, a child might be observed playing at home with familiar toys. During observations of this manner, the child may not even be aware that others are watching. A slightly more structured approach might include a child being presented with a specific set of toys or objects, with the observations taking place in a room specifically arranged for such a purpose. There are advantages as well as disadvantages to each of these approaches. Naturalistic observations afford the EI an opportunity to examine play free from imposed structure. This allows evaluation of how a child responds to varying contexts. Naturalistic evaluations can be conducted virtually any time or any place with few additional resources needed besides the observer. The lack of structure and predictability inherent in less organized observations of play may be a source of concern for the EI. However, many EIs are using free-play situations in the form of arena evaluations to elicit wide samples of infant and child performance.

A second strategy to assess play involves a more structured format for the elicitation of behaviors. This procedure elicits behaviors through modeling and/or verbal description of the performance a child is to demonstrate. The child may be presented with a series of objects and asked to demonstrate various activities. For example, the child may be given a doll and a brush and be asked to brush the doll's hair. Or the child may be given a doll and a brush, with the examiner demonstrating brushing the doll's hair followed by a request that the child demonstrate the identical activity.

Westby (1980) presented information about the assessment of cognitive and communication ability through play. The Westby data linked play behaviors with concurrent communication skills that should be observed at various ages. A sample of the play activities and the concurrent communication behaviors expected at each age is presented in Table 3–9. Although the concept of measuring play is

TABLE 3-9 Symbolic Play Scale Checklist

Play Activity	Communication Activity
Stage I: 9–12 Months	
Awareness that objects exist when not seen	No true language; may have words associated with some actions
Does not mouth or bang all toys	Exhibits some command and request behaviors
Stage II: 13–17 Months	
Purposeful exploration of toys; discovers operation of toys through trial and error	Single words used (context dependent); communicative functions include request, command, response, greeting, protesting
Hands toy to adult if unable to operate on own	
Stage III: 17–19 Months	
Child pretends to go to sleep or drink from cup	Beginning of true verbal communication
Stage IV: 19–22 Months	
Symbolic play extends beyond the child's self	Beginning of word combinations with following semantic relations
Child plays with dolls, combines two toys in play, performs pretend activities	
Stage V: 24 Months	
Represents daily experiences, plays house, uses objects in a realistic manner	Increased use of phrases and short sentences
	Following morphologic markers appear: "ing" endings, plurals, possessives
Stage VI: 30 Months	
Represents events less frequently experienced	Responds to WH questions: who, what, whose, where
	Asks WH questions
Stage VII: 36 Months	
Obvious sequence to play activities	Uses past tense
Associative play	Uses future aspects (particularly "gonna") such as "I'm gonna wash dishes."

Adapted from "Assessment of Language and Cognitive Abilities through Play," by C. Westby, 1980, *Language and Hearing Services in the Schools, 3*, p. 154.

relatively new, information such as that provided by Westby assists the EI in using play measurements as part of an overall assessment of communication skills. Numerous consistencies exist between play and communication performance. Change in play complexity is generally accompanied by changes in communication status. It is precisely these changes that form the basis for the assessment of play.

Assessment of Pragmatics

Pragmatics is the use of language in social contexts and includes the rules that govern how language is used for communication. Three different levels of pragmatics are generally described. These are intentions, conversational discourse, and role taking. Each of these will be discussed briefly in the information following.

Intentions

Communicative intentions are the rationale behind an individual using language to communicate. There is general progression in communicative intentions in developing children. This progression moves from prelinguistic to one-word to multiword expressions of intentions. During the earliest months of a child's life, unintentional signals are sent to caregivers. These include indications of discomfort, fear, anxiety, and pleasure. Although unintentional, adults may interpret them as intentional. Later, the child demonstrates nonverbal behaviors that more readily reflect intentional communication. These are more readily interpreted by adults as purposeful. These behaviors may include requests for objects, attention seeking, and protesting. Later, at approximately 12 to 15 months of age, these same intentions are expressed through the use of words. The child may combine gesture with words and readily repeats messages not understood by adults. Roberts and Crais (1989) describe a variety of behaviors that characterize communication intentions frequently expressed by children at the prelinguistic, one-word, and multiword stages (Table 3–10). It is possible to measure the manner in which intentions are expressed by children during these early stages of communication development.

Discourse

The second area that relates to pragmatics is discourse. For a child to be able to interact with others, he or she must learn how to participate

TABLE 3-10 Communication Intentions Expressed in Prelinguistic, One-Word, and Multiword Utterances

Intention	Prelinguistic	One-Word	Multiword
Attention seeking	Child tugs on mother's skirt	Says "mommy" as tugs	Says "You know what?"
Requests object	Child points to toy	Says name of toy	Says "Give me the ____."
Requests action	Child places adult's hand on desired object	Says word to identify desired action	Tells adult what action is desired
Protest	Pushes adult's hand away when undesired food is offered	Says "no" in response to undesired food	Says "No peas mama."
Greeting	Child waves as mother leaves	Says "Bye."	Says "Bye mom."

Adapted from "Assessing Communicative Skills" (p. 310), by J. Roberts and E. Crais in *Assessing Infants and Preschoolers with Handicaps*, edited by D. Bailey and M. Wolery, 1989, Columbus, OH: Merrill.

in a conversation. In other words, the child must become a conversationalist. This refers to how the individual learns to initiate and exit a conversation, take turns, and move from one topic to another. To participate in a conversation, a child must learn these rules. If the child chooses to initiate a conversation, he must follow a logical progression that includes eliciting the listener's attention, speaking clearly, providing sufficient information so that the listener can identify the topic, and providing sufficient information to allow the listener to identify appropriate relations between words. An additional skill that must be learned is that of topic maintenance spanning several conversational turns. A child must learn to identify the need to take turns, the length of the turn, how to take a turn, when it is appropriate to take a turn, as well as when it is unacceptable to take a turn. These skills are essential for a child because discourse skills are integral to effective communication. Without these conversational skills, the child's communicative ability is limited.

Role Taking

Role taking is generally described as the third area of pragmatics. Role taking is a child's ability to take the perspective of the listener during conversation. The child must learn to monitor what the listener is comprehending, and act accordingly. This means that the child must learn to direct attention toward not only what is being said but also what a listener understands. If the child perceives that the message is not fully comprehended by the listener, modifications in the content or manner of the communication must take place. More intricate role-taking skills in the context of pragmatic development do not take place until the later elementary school years.

In any area of development that is linked to maturational changes, measurement is possible. This is true of pragmatic development as well. Antoniadis, Didow, Lockhart, and Moroge (1984) present information on screening for early cognitive and communication behaviors. In the information provided, direction relative to screening for pragmatic development is included. Normative data is not included. However, the basic details afford the EI a framework for making structured observations of social-pragmatic use in infants and toddlers. Table 3–11 presents a sample of the behaviors included in the scale. Several existing infant-toddler communication assessment tools incorporate the measurement of pragmatic skills into their overall measure of communication status.

TABLE 3–11 Social Communication Pragmatics Screening Items

Age (Months)	Behaviors
0–9	Intracommunicative behaviors such as cry, touch, smile, vocalize, grasp, suck, laugh
0–9	Reciprocal gesture
9–18	Demonstrates communicative intent by pointing to objects, showing objects, giving objects
9–18	Regulates behavior of self and others
9–18	Protests (voice or gesture)
9–18	Develops verbal turn taking
18–24	Engages in adultlike dialogue
18–24	Uses language to pretend
18–24	Uses language to control and interact with others

Adapted from "Screening for Early Cognitive and Communicative Behaviors," by A. Antoniadis, S. Didow, S. Lockhart, and P. Morogue, 1984, *Communique, 9*, p. 14.

Assessment of Gesture

The use of gesture by children under 3 years of age is known to be preliminary to verbal communication. Hence, it is possible for the EI to make structured observations of gestural usage by the child. A variety of formats can be used to observe gesture development. In addition, many existing assessment instruments incorporate gesture as part of the assessment strategy. Normative data regarding gestural development is limited. However, ample data (gestural) exists that can be used by the EI as part of a comprehensive evaluation of communication skills.

Olswang, Stoel-Gammons, Coggins, and Carpenter (1987) have provided one of the better instruments incorporating measurements of gesture. Gesture behaviors are listed in six distinct categories, and the EI simply indicates whether a particular behavior is present. The six categories are (1) social regulation and social games; (2) greeting, signs of affection, and bedtime; (3) eating and drinking; (4) dressing, grooming, and washing; (5) adult activities; and (6) toys and games. A sample of the specific behaviors included in the gesture inventory is provided in Table 3–12. The information provided in the appendix at the end of this chapter lists several communication assessment instruments that incorporate gesture into an overall paradigm of assessment.

TABLE 3-12   *Gesture Inventory Behaviors*

Social Regulation and Social Games
   "Up" (arms reaching upward in request to be picked up)
   Showing (extends arm toward other with object in hand)
   Peek-a-boo (covers and uncovers face)
   "All gone" (shrugs and puts out hands in gesture of surprise)

Greetings, Signs of Affection
   Waves hi/bye
   Hugs (dolls, people, animals)
   Puts to bed (puts dolls, people, or animals to bed)
   Rocks (dolls, people, or animals)

Eating and Drinking
   Drinking (places container to mouth)
   Feeding others (puts utensil to mouth of others/doll)
   Wipes (wipes hands or face with napkin or bib)
   Pouring (makes gesture of pouring from container)

Dressing, Grooming, and Washing
   Combs or brushes hair
   Brushes teeth
   Hat (puts on or tries to put on)
   Diapering (takes off/puts on diaper, powders bottom)

Adult Activities
   Telephone (puts receiver to ear)
   Pushes stroller or shopping cart
   Musical instrument (tries to play an instrument)
   Writing or typing

Toys and Games
   Ball (throws or kicks ball)
   Car/truck (rolls or pushes toy vehicle)
   Gun/pistol (makes a shooting gesture)
   Airplane (makes a gesture of flying a plane or helicopter)

Adapted from *Assessing Linguistic Behaviors* (p. 1), by L. Olswang, C. Stoel-Gammons, T. Coggins, and R. Carpenter, 1987, Seattle, WA: University of Washington Press.

Although there is overlap between the behaviors of gesture and play, this is not necessarily negative. Rather, it alerts the EI to the need to comprehensively monitor all behaviors reflective of a child's developing communicative competence.

Assessment of Language Comprehension and Expression

As has been previously noted, age-appropriate communication skill is the single best predictor of school performance. Hence, comprehensive monitoring of language skills, particularly as a child approaches school age, is imperative. When one recalls that communication is the developmental domain that with greatest frequency distinguishes at-risk from low-risk or no-risk children, the monitoring of communication skills takes on even greater importance. Coplan (1985) reinforces this view by noting that in the course of a normal day the busy pediatrician will see at least one or two children with communication delay. Given the prevalence of communication delay in children from birth to 3 years of age, it is mandatory that the EI become familiar with procedures for assessing overall communication skills and, in particular, language comprehension and expression. The information to follow is not intended as an exhaustive review of language comprehension and expression assessment. Rather, it is designed to alert the EI to issues related to effective appraisal of these important skills.

Language Comprehension

A strong link between cognition, comprehension, and production of language exists. As children demonstrate maturational changes in their communicative status, behaviors that display such change should be evident and, therefore, measurable. Hence, it is precisely behaviors of this nature that form the basis for measuring language comprehension status.

Few available instruments are used solely as language comprehension tools. Rather, language comprehension is generally measured as part of a more comprehensive assessment of overall communication skills and performance. Assessment of language comprehension must focus on a child's ability to comprehend language apart from nonlinguistic cues. Although several assessment tools are mentioned at the end of this chapter, it is imperative that the EI be alert to all behaviors that may be reflective of a child's comprehension ability. As such, all actions indicating the child's ability to comprehend meaning are of interest to the EI. One helpful suggestion is provided by Paul and Fischer (1985). They suggest that the examiner briefly interview caregivers by telephone regarding a child's comprehension competence. This affords the EI an opportunity to gather important indexes of the child's comprehension ability before administration of a formal assessment tool and apart from the pitfalls inherent in formal assessment procedures. A communication-based parent interview format is provided by Rossetti (1990a).

Rowan and Johnson (1988) describe an assessment procedure that is designed to monitor language comprehension for children birth through 12 months of age. The procedure lists specific behaviors thought to reflect comprehension competence. Parental report, examiner observations, and observations made during direct testing are all applicable. Table 3–13 presents a sampling of comprehension items by age.

If the EI chooses to use a formal assessment tool in monitoring language comprehension skill, the process is simplified somewhat. This is because such a tool will trace comprehension skills in a manner that adequately reflects normal comprehension development. However, if a less formal approach is used, it is imperative that the EI become familiar with normal development of language comprehension skills for children birth through 3 years of age. The overall procedure involves the establishment of a baseline of comprehension mastery followed by the assessment of more complicated comprehension capacity. This procedure is continued until a ceiling of comprehension ability is established.

Chapman (1981) has provided a helpful format for monitoring language comprehension ability. Table 3–14 presents an overview of the Chapman approach. As Chapman suggests, comprehension of single words without the support of nonlinguistic cues indicates performance expected in the age range of 12 to 18 months. If the child is unable to demonstrate performance in this manner, request may be accompanied by gesture. Achievement in this manner implies comprehension ability in the age range of 8 to 12 months. Once basic comprehension is established at the 12- to 18-month level, more difficult comprehension tasks may be introduced. A developmental progression of comprehension skills is followed. This includes understanding of two-word instructions. Both familiar and unfamiliar combinations of words can be used when the EI is attempting to monitor comprehension at the 18- to 24-month level. After 24 months of age, a broader array of formal assessment instruments is available for use in measuring language comprehension ability. The collection of samples of behavior during assessment should be supported in all instances with data gathered from careful interview of caregivers.

Accurate assessment of language comprehension ability involves considerable skill on the part of the EI. Regardless of primary academic discipline, it is imperative that all EI personnel familiarize themselves as broadly as possible with issues related to language development and performance. It is precisely this base of information that will prove invaluable as the process of communication assessment unfolds.

TABLE 3–13 Language Comprehension Items by Age

Age (Months)	Comprehension Item
0–3	
_____	Alerting response to sound
_____	Activity diminishes or ceases when approached by sound
_____	Quieted by familiar voice
_____	Smiles at mother's voice
_____	Often watches speaker's mouth
3–6	
_____	Shows fear of angry voice
_____	Anticipates feeding at sight of food
_____	Recognizes and responds to name
_____	Appears to recognize words like "up" and "bye-bye"
_____	Responds to pleasant speech by smiling
6–9	
_____	Moves toward or searches for family member when named
_____	Begins to show recognition of "no"
_____	Begins to anticipate visual games
_____	Shows stranger anxiety
_____	Relates sound to object
9–12	
_____	Action response to verbal request
_____	Shakes head yes or no
_____	Understands "hot" and "so big"
_____	Understands some action words
_____	Frowns when scolded
_____	May follow simple commands when given by gesture

Adapted from "Screening and Assessment," by L. Rowan and C. Johnson, 1988 (June), paper presented at Infant and Toddler Communication Workshop, Minneapolis, MN.

Language Expression

The overall incidence of language delay in childhood ranges from 3% to 15%, depending on the criteria one wishes to use in defining language delay. Of all preschool children ages 3 to 5 who are identified as disabled, 70% have speech and language impairments (Prizant, Weatherby, & Roberts, 1993). Hence, disorders of communication are

TABLE 3–14　Language Comprehension Ability by Age

Age (months)	Comprehension Ability	Comprehension Strategy
8–12	Understands a few single words in routine context	1. Looks at objects mother looks at 2. Acts on objects noticed 3. Imitates ongoing action
12–18	Understands single words; outside of routine, some contextual cues needed	1. Attends to object mentioned 2. Performs usual activities with familiar objects
18–24	Understands words for absent objects; some two-word combinations understood	1. Locates objects mentioned 2. Follows simple commands
24–36	Comprehension of three-word sentences; needs context of past experience to determine meaning	1. Supplies missing information

Adapted from "Exploring Children's Communicative Intents" (p. 22), by R. Chapman in *Assessing Language Production in Children: Experimental Procedures*, edited by J. Miller, 1981, Baltimore: University Park Press.

the most common developmental disability in children. Approximately 1% of the pediatric population will display severe language delay. Long-term outcome for children with milder language delay is variable, with the majority displaying persistent language problems as well as more general cognitive and learning problems (Capute & Accardo, 1991). It is easy, from information such as this, to perceive the need for early identification of language delay and, more specifically, expressive language impairment.

Effective assessment of expressive language ability involves more than a simple accounting of the number of words in a child's expressive vocabulary or the average number of words contained in a child's expressive utterances. Although these issues are of importance in assessing expressive communication skills, they do not constitute the primary focus of assessment. Table 3–15 presents a checklist of expected expressive behaviors by age. Assessment instruments designed to monitor expressive language development must use data of this nature in assessing expressive language performance.

Regardless of which assessment procedures are employed (test administration, communication sampling, or both), initial assessment considerations must include measurement of communicative means (the behaviors by which information is communicated) and communicative functions (the purposes for which a child communicates). In addition, assessment of the behaviors of a child's communicative partners is important. Communicative partners include people who interact with a child on a regular basis. Partners may both support the child's communicative competence or hinder overall growth in communicative skills. Communication-based intervention, as discussed in later chapters, is heavily dependent on involving the caregivers in the child's intervention program. Hence, it is imperative that some indication of the status of the child's interaction with communicative partners be made.

A helpful manner in which to view communication assessment for children under 3 years is presented by Roth (1990). The first distinction that Roth suggests is that the EI note whether the child uses socialized or nonsocialized communication. Speech that is addressed to a listener is considered socialized speech (communication). It presupposes an obligation on the part of the listener to respond in some manner. Another example of socialized communication is verbal play, which involves mutual engagement between communicative partners. It includes turn taking and contingent response patterns. Socialized communication differs from nonsocialized communication in that the latter is not directed toward a listener and no response is required. This type of communication may include monologues,

TABLE 3–15 Checklist of Expected Expressive Communication Behavior

By 6 Months
1. Vocalizes any sound
2. Produces range of vocalizations
3. Produces a variety of facial expressions

By 12 Months
1. Babbles with variety of consonant-like sounds
2. Takes turns vocalizing
3. Imitates vocalizations or gestures
4. Uses conventional gestures (points) and vocalizations
5. Communicates for behavior regulation, social interaction, and joint attention

By 18 Months
1. Produces a variety of sounds that may sound like words or short sentences
2. Uses variety of gestures and vocalizations to request objects and direct attention
3. Produces a few meaningful words

By 24 Months
1. Uses at least 10 to 15 words meaningfully
2. Uses two-word sentences meaningfully, including simple sentences
3. Speech is present and at least 50% intelligible to caregivers

By 36 Months
1. Produces sentences of 3 to 5 words
2. Talks about past and future events
3. Asks questions using "what," "who," and "where"
4. Has vocabulary of 100 to 200 words; speech is greater than 75% intelligible to caregivers

Adapted from "Communication Disorders in Infants and Toddlers" (p. 260), by B. Prizant, A. Weatherby, and J. Roberts in *Handbook of Infant Mental Health*, edited by C. Zeanah, 1993, New York: Guilford Press.

songs, rhymes, and various sounds made during play. Although socialized speech may result from communication that was intended as nonsocial initially, no response is needed by the child. Assessment of the child's expressive ability may include a determination of the proportion of the child's communication that fits into each category. Information of this type is typically gained through free-play interactions with the child. Although no specific norms exist for the proportion of communication that should be socialized versus nonsocialized by age, the EI is encouraged to pay attention to these two basic categories of communicative situations.

Turn taking is an important measure of the child's expressive communication status. There is significant information suggesting that mother-infant interactions involve turn taking very early in the mother-infant relationship (perhaps as early as shortly after birth). This process is initially set in motion through a child's experience with his or her mother. Infants are uniquely attuned to the human face and voice from the earliest hours of life. Thus, it is no surprise that the mother and child, in a relatively short period of time, learn how to communicate with each other (synchrony). These communications are characterized by turn taking. Communicative initiations are generally initiated by the child, but the adult may prolong the turn-taking exchanges. Later (after 4 to 7 months of age), the child and adult may initiate and prolong turn-taking exchanges with equal frequency. Turn taking is also observed in the repetitive games and routines between mother and child. Social routines (peek-a-boo, how big is baby, and so on) become important vehicles that engage the child's attention in learning how to take turns as the communication becomes more complex in nature. It is important that the EI observe any social ritual games (rich in communication and turn taking) that may be part of the child's normal caregiving routine. The EI is encouraged to monitor turn taking as part of an overall assessment of expressive communication skills.

In addition to turn taking, conversational initiation is a sensitive indicator of expressive communication skills. When measuring communication initiations, the EI needs to be interested in determining whether the child initiates conversational topics, how these conversations are initiated, and the outcome (success or failure) of the child's initiation attempts. Foster (1986) presents a developmental sequence of topic initiation skills for children between 1 month and 2.5 years of age. This information is presented in a developmental sequence of three stages. The first stage is self topics. This stage involves unintentional or deliberate messages conveyed by the neonate to the adult. These may include messages of illness or a hunger cry. Toward the end of the first year, the initiations expand to include environmental topics. These are things in the child's immediate environment. By the middle of the second year, the child will demonstrate communication initiations that include such abstract topics as where objects come from and something the child anticipates doing in the future.

Once communicative initiations are established, the child must learn to demonstrate conversational maintenance. Maintenance of a topic during a conversation is generally dependent on the response the child receives for a preceding message. Without this skill, true conversation is impossible even if proper turns are taken. Conversation maintenance may take one of two forms. One pattern reflects a simple maintenance of the topic, with the second pattern being maintenance of the topic and the addition of new information as part of the conversation. Although the first pattern may lead to topic maintenance, the second pattern has a greater likelihood of keeping the conversation going for a longer period of time and for more turns between child and adult. Data from several sources suggests that adult-child conversations tend to be maintained over a large number of turns when the child initiates the topic and when the focus of the conversation is an object present in the child's world. As part of the measurement process for conversational maintenance, both verbal and nonverbal messages focused on a single topic must be identified. This can be a difficult task because conversations change rapidly midstream. However, the EI must be alert to strategies designed to enhance the measurement of turn taking and topic maintenance.

How children handle breakdowns in conversations may also be a valuable assessment target. If a conversation breakdown is not repaired by the adult or the child, the result is a communication failure. Younger children do not readily attempt to repair broken conversations. At approximately 2 years of age, the beginning of conversational repair may be observed. For a more complete discussion of conversational repair, see Gallagher and Darnton (1978).

CHAPTER SUMMARY

As is readily apparent from the information presented in this chapter, effective assessment of socio-communicative skills is a significantly more involved process than simply administering an assessment instrument. Assessment of socio-communication skills is not a product, but rather a process. The process is designed to enhance the EI's understanding of the child's communicative competencies and resources. As such, assessment should be an ongoing, collaborative process of systematic observation and analysis. The process involves formulating questions, gathering information from multiple sources, sharing observations, and making interpretations in order to form new questions ("Toward a New Vision," 1994).

In *Zero to Three* (1994), the results of a Working Group on Developmental Assessment are presented. The working group presents a list of guiding principles that should be kept in mind as assessment services are delivered to children birth through 3 years of age. These guidelines are presented in summary form as follows:

1. Assessment must be based on an integrated developmental model. This suggests that the full complexity of the child's development must be considered as assessment services are provided.

2. Assessment must involve multiple sources of information and multiple components. This suggests that no one source of information regarding the child's socio-communicative competence is more important than another.

3. The child's relationship and interactions with his or her most trusted caregiver should form the cornerstone of the assessment. Spontaneous, motivated interactions between a child and caregiver provide an optimal setting for a good sample of the child's behavior.

4. Assessment should identify the child's current level of functioning (strengths), as well as additional competencies the child needs to develop to attain additional landmarks which represent developmental progress. This suggests that a functional interpretation of skill status is best, rather than statements suggesting that a child is a certain number of months behind normal developmental expectations.

5. Assessment is a collaborative process. This implies that assessment involves ongoing collaboration between clinicians and parents.

6. The process of assessment should always be viewed as the first step in a potential intervention process. Assessment is not an end in itself. Rather, it is the starting point for further activities designed to enhance the child's performance level.

7. Young children should never be challenged by assessment by a strange examiner. The best samples of behavior on which to base developmental status are made when the child feels safe and comfortable.

8. Assessments that are limited to areas that are easily measurable, such as certain motor or cognitive skills, should not be considered complete. Assessment tools that are used simply because they are available or because staff are trained to use them are generally inadequate. Such assessments are inadequate because they do not provide an integrated understanding of the child's performance. Further,

they generally do not measure the child's capacities as manifested in spontaneous interactions with caregivers.

9. Formal tests or tools should not be the cornerstone of the assessment of an infant or young child. The behaviors collected during formal test administration are only approximations of the child's true functional abilities. Tests and instruments are not designed or able to bring out the child's unique ability and potential.

These principles embody a philosophy of infant-toddler assessment that is in agreement with the precepts contained in this chapter. All the information contained in this chapter is designed to expand the EI's arsenal of assessment skills. The outcome will be more accurate and reliable assessment data, resulting in effective and reliable intervention activity.

REFERENCES

Ainsworth, M., Blehar, M., Waters, E., & Wall, S. (1978). *Patterns of attachment: A psychological study of the strange situation.* Hillsdale, NJ: Lawrence Erlbaum Associates.

Antoniadis, A., Didow, S., Lockhart, S., & Morogue, P. (1984). Screening for early cognitive and communicative behaviors. *Communique, 9,* 14.

Bond, L., Creasy, G., & Abrams, C. (1990). Play assessment: Reflecting and promoting cognitive competence. In E. Gibbs & D. Teti (Eds.), *Interdisciplinary assessment of infants: A guide for early intervention professionals* (p. 382). Baltimore: Paul H. Brookes.

Brazelton, T. (1973). *Neonatal behavior assessment scale.* Philadelphia: J. B. Lippincott.

Capute, A., & Accardo, P. (1991). Language assessment. In A. Capute & P. Accardo (Eds.), *Developmental disabilities in infancy and childhood* (p. 29). Baltimore: Paul H. Brookes.

Casby, M. (1992). Symbolic play: Development and assessment considerations. *Infants and Young Children, 4,* 43.

Chapman, R. (1981). Exploring children's communicative intents. In J. Miller (Ed.), *Assessing language production in children: Experimental procedures* (p. 11). Baltimore: University Park Press.

Coggins, T. (1991). Bringing context back into assessment. *Topics in Language Disorders, 11,* 43.

Coplan, J. (1982). Parental estimate of child's developmental level in a high risk population. *American Journal of Disorders in Childhood, 136,* 101.

Coplan, J. (1985). Evaluation of the child with delayed speech or language. *Pediatric Annals, 14,* 3.

Farran, D., Clark, K., & Ray, A. (1990). Measures of parent-child interaction. In E. Gibbs & D. Teti (Eds.), *Interdisciplinary assessment of infants: A guide for early intervention professionals* (p. 210). Baltimore: Paul H. Brookes.

Filler, J. (1983). Service models for handicapped infants. In S. Gray Garwood & R. Fewell (Eds.), *Educating handicapped infants* (p. 290). Rockville, MD: Aspen Publications.

Foley, G. (1990). Portrait of an arena evaluation: Assessment in the transdisciplinary approach. In E. Gibbs & D. Teti (Eds.), *Transdisciplinary assessment of infants* (p. 310). Baltimore: Paul H. Brookes.

Foster, S. (1986). Learning discourse topic maintenance in the preschool years. *Journal of Child Language, 13*, 231.

Gallagher, T., & Darnton, B. (1978). Conversational aspects of the speech of language-disordered children: Revision behaviors. *Journal of Speech and Hearing Disorders, 21*, 118.

Gorski, P., Davidson, M., & Brazelton, T. (1979). Stages of behavioral organization in the high risk neonate: Theoretical and clinical considerations. *Seminars in Perinatology, 3*, 61.

Haynes, U. (1983). *Holistic health care for children with disabilities*. Baltimore: University Park Press.

Hutt, M., Menninger, W., & O'Keefe, D. (1947). The neuropsychiatric team in the United States Army. *Mental Health, 31*, 103.

Jacobsen, C., Starnes, C., & Gasser, V. (1988). An experimental analysis of the generalization of description and praises for mothers of premature infants. *Human Communication, 12*, 23.

Klaus, M., & Kennell, J. (1976). *Maternal-infant bonding*. St. Louis, MO: C. V. Mosby.

Klein, D., & Briggs, M. (1986). *Observation of communication interaction scoring sheet (OCI). Observation of communication interaction: A model program to facilitate positive communication interactions between caregivers and their high-risk infants* (DHHS Publication No. MCJ 06351-01-0). Washington, DC: U.S. Government Printing Office.

Largo, R., Molinari, L., Pinto, L., & Weber, M. (1986). Language development of term and preterm children during the first five years of life. *Developmental Medicine and Child Neurology, 28*, 333.

Linder, T. (1993). *Transdisciplinary play-based assessment: A functional approach to working with young children*. Baltimore: Paul H. Brookes.

McCarthy, J. (1980). Assessment of young children with learning problems: Beyond the paralysis of analysis. In E. Sell (Ed.), *Follow-up of the high-risk newborn: A practical approach* (p. 59). Springfield, IL: Charles C. Thomas.

McCormick, M., Shapiro, S., & Starfield, B. (1982). Factors associated with maternal opinion of infant development: Clues to the vulnerable child. *Pediatrics, 69*, 537.

Mindes, G. (1982). Social and cognitive aspects of play in young handicapped children. *Topics in Early Childhood Special Education, 2*, 14.

Murphy, T., Nichter, C., & Liden, C. (1982). Developmental outcome of the high risk infant: A review of methodological issues. *Seminars in Perinatology, 6*, 4.

Olswang, L., Stoel-Gammon, C., Coggins, T., & Carpenter, R. (1987). *Assessing linguistic behaviors*. Seattle, WA: University of Washington Press.

Palisano, R., Short, M., & Nelson, D. (1985). Chronological age vs. adjusted age in assessing motor development of healthy twelve month old premature and full-term infants. *Physical and Occupational Therapy in Pediatrics, 5*, 1.

Paul, R., & Fischer, M. (1985, November). *Sentence comprehension strategies in children with autism and developmental language disorders.* Paper presented at the Symposium for Research in Child Language Disorders, Madison, WI.

Prizant, B., Weatherby, A., & Roberts, J. (1993). Communication disorders in infants and toddlers. In C. Zeanah (Ed.), *Handbook of infant mental health* (p. 260). New York: Guilford Press.

Rescorla, L. (1991). Identifying expressive language delay at age two. *Topics in Language Disorders, 11*, 14.

Roberts, J., & Crais, E. (1989). Assessing communication skills. In D. Bailey & M. Wolery (Eds.), *Assessing infants and preschoolers with handicaps* (p. 98). Columbus, OH: Merrill.

Rossetti, L. (1990a). *Infant-toddler assessment: An interdisciplinary approach.* Boston: Little, Brown & Company.

Rossetti, L. (1990b). *The Rossetti infant-toddler language scale. A measure of communication and interaction.* East Moline, IL: LinguiSystems.

Roth, F. (1990). Early language assessment. In E. Gibbs & D. Teti (Eds.), *Interdisciplinary assessment of infants: A guide for early intervention professionals* (p. 200). Baltimore: Paul H. Brookes.

Rowan, L., & Johnson, C. (1988, June). *Screening and assessment.* Paper presented at the Infant and Toddler Communication and Assessment Workshop, Minneapolis, MN.

Siegel, L. (1983). Correction for prematurity and its consequences for the assessment of the very low birth weight infant. *Child Development, 54*, 1174.

Sparks, S. (1989). Assessment and intervention with at-risk infants and toddlers: Guidelines for the speech-language pathologist. *Topics in Language Disorders, 10*, 43.

Sparks, S., Clark, M., Oas, D., & Erickson, R. (1988, November). *Clinical services to infants at risk for communication disorders.* Paper presented at the annual convention of the American Speech-Language-Hearing Association, Boston.

Terrell, B., & Schwartz, R. (1988). Object transformation in the play of language impaired children. *Journal of Speech and Hearing Disorders, 53*, 459.

Teti, D., & Nakagawa, M. (1990). Assessing attachment in infancy. In E. Gibbs & D. Teti (Eds.), *Interdisciplinary assessment of infants: A guide for early intervention professionals* (p. 310). Baltimore: Paul H. Brookes.

Theadore, G., Maher, S., & Prizant, B. (1990). Early assessment and intervention with emotional and behavioral disorders and communication disorders. *Topics in Language Disorders, 10*, 42.

Toward a new vision for the developmental assessment of infants and young children. (1994). *Zero to Three, 14*, 1.

U.S. Department of Education. Twelfth annual report to the Congress on the implementation of the Education of the Handicapped Act. (1990). Washington, DC.

Walker, L., & Thompson, E. (1982). Mother-infant play interaction scale. In S. Humenick-Smith (Ed.), *Analysis of current assessment strategies in the health care of young children and childbearing families* (p. 56). Norwich, CT: Williams & Wilkins.

Westby, C. (1980). Assessment of language and cognitive abilities through play. *Language and Hearing Services in the Schools, 3,* 154.

APPENDIX 3 A: SELECTED INFANT-TODDLER ASSESSMENT INSTRUMENTS

Measures of Infant-Caregiver Interaction and Attachment

Barnard Teaching Scale and Barnard Feeding Scale

Nursing Child Assessment Satellite Training (NCAST). (1978). Nursing Child Assessment Feeding Scale. (Manual available during training with NCAST trainers. Contact Georgina Sumner, NCAST, WJ-10, University of Washington, Seattle, WA 98195).

The teaching and feeding scales (also known as the NCAST) use two structured situations for measuring caregiver and child behaviors. The goal of the scales is to identify factors that may be predictive of later child development. The caregiver scale measures four specific areas, which include sensitivity to cues, response to child's distress, social-emotional growth fostering, and cognitive growth fostering. Two areas are measured for the child: clarity of cues and responsiveness to caregiver. The scale is not simple to administer, and specific training is required for proper use.

Greenspan-Lieberman Observation System for Assessment of Caregiver-Infant Interaction During Semi-Structured Play

Greenspan, S., & Poisson, S. (1983). Greenspan-Lieberman Observation System for Assessment of Caregiver-Infant Interaction during Semi-Structured Play (GLOS). Division of Maternal and Child Health, HRSA, DHHS, Rockville, MD 20850.

The primary goal of this system was to develop an instrument that defined observable and measurable behaviors and that can be used clinically in assessing mother-infant interactions. The scale is based on three premises. The first is that the infant is capable of adaptive responses to the environment from birth. The second premise is that this behavior becomes more organized during the first two years. The third is that infants show individual differences from the time of birth and that those differences are related to later development of coping skills. The system consists of careful evaluation of videotaped samples of interactions between caregiver and infant in a laboratory setting. Four versions are currently available: the newborn scale, the infant scale, the toddler scale, and the 3-year-old version. One primary criticism of the system is the nature of the scoring system employed, and the setting in which the samples are obtained. It is generally preferred that samples of mother-infant interaction take place in as naturalistic a setting as possible. The system is a large and complicated tool that may find less acceptance among busy early intervention professionals.

Interpersonal Behavior Constructs (IBC)

Kogan, K., & Gordon, B. (1975). A mother-instruction program: Documenting change in mother-child interactions. *Child Psychiatry and Human Development, 5,* 189.

The IBC was developed for the purpose of observing, analyzing, and delineating unique patterns and styles of mother-child interactions within a broad behavioral framework. The IBC views the child's behavior as being under the primary control of the immediate social environment; the social relationship between caregiver and child is viewed as bidirectional. The IBC provides information regarding changes in parental and child interactive behaviors following a behaviorally focused intervention program. The behaviors collected and analyzed contribute information about the quality of caregiver-child interactions.

Maternal Behavior Rating Scale (MBRS)

Mahoney, G., Powell, A., & Finger, I. (1986). The Maternal Behavior Rating Scale. *Topics in Early Childhood Special Education, 6,* 44.

The MBRS was developed for the purpose of assessing the impact of early intervention services upon the quality of maternal interactive behavior; it is designed to be used with videotaped home observations of free-play interactions between mother and child. The targeted populations are mother-child dyads in which the children are diagnosed with medical or physiological conditions associated with mental retardation. The authors wanted to identify patterns of maternal behavior that are related to different levels of children's development. The MBRS rates 18 maternal behaviors on a 5-point Likert scale. Definitions for maternal behaviors and anchors for the 5-point rating are provided in the scale manual. Four child behaviors are related also.

Parent Behavior Progression (PBP)

Allen, D., Affleck, G., McQueeny, M., & McGrade, B. (1982). Validation of the Parent Behavior Progression in early intervention programs. *Mental Retardation, 20,* 159.

The PBP was developed to be appropriate for observation following two or three home visits with a mother and a low-birth-weight or premature infant for the purpose of assessing maternal behaviors from which short-term goals may be formulated. Parental behaviors are viewed as forming a six-level progression. Parents need not acquire behaviors at one level before they progress to the next level. Specific behaviors are checked within each level as either present or absent. The first three levels establish an affective base that is believed to promote attachment. Levels 4 to 6 involve experiences that will optimize the infant's cognitive development. There are two forms available: one for children below 9 months of age and another for children 9 to 36 months of age. One major criticism of this system is that the scoring is less well defined than most observers might prefer. Another difficulty arises in using the results as a tool for planning intervention and monitoring progress because behaviors at lower levels need not be acquired before behaviors at later levels.

Parent/Caregiver Involvement Scale (PCIS)

Farran, D., Kasari, C., Jay, S., & Comfort, M. (1986). Parent/Caregiver Involvement Scale. (Available from Continuing Education, University of North Carolina at Greensboro, Greensboro, NC 27413).

The PCIS is organized into 11 behaviors that are rated on three dimensions: amount, quality, and developmental appropriateness. Each behavior on the scale is rated on a 5-point scale with odd-numbered points behaviorally anchored. Ratings of a series of maternal behaviors in videotaped free-play interactions in a laboratory setting are used. The scale is used for children 3 to 36 months of age and has been adapted for home or clinic use. It has also been constructed for use with infants with special needs and their mothers. The behaviors that are rated are presumed to be necessary for the child's cognitive growth and feelings of self-esteem. The overall presumption of the scale is that adults are important mediators of experience for the child, bridging between the child's immaturity/inexperience and interactions with objects and ideas in the world. The scale provides a comprehensive description of caregiver interactions with infants and can be a helpful source of information for EI providers as part of a comprehensive assessment of adult caregiving styles and ability.

Strange Situation Procedure (SSP)

Ainsworth, M., Blehar, M., Waters, E., & Wall, S. (1978). *Patterns of attachment: A psychological study of the strange situation.* Hillsdale, NJ: Lawrence Erlbaum Associates.

The SSP is designed to identity infant behaviors that represent anxiety when presented with a novel or strange situation, one new to the infant. It has been used primarily as a research tool and not as extensively to identify infants who might be "insecurely attached" to their primary caregiver. In other words, some of the behaviors measured may not be completely reliable as indicators of difficulty in caregiver-infant attachment. The SSP assesses attachment security by examining changes in the attachment exploration balance as it relates to changes in factors external to the infant. The SSP should not be used as the sole measure of attachment, but rather in concert with additional procedures designed to monitor caregiver-infant attachment.

Attachment Q-Set

Waters, E., & Deane, K. (1985). Defining and assessing individual differences in attachment relationships: Q-methodology and the organization of behavior in infancy and early childhood. In I. Bretherton & E. Waters (Eds.), Growing points of attachment theory and research. *Monographs of the Society for Research in Child Development, 50,* 41.

The Attachment Q-Set is composed of 90 behavioral descriptions that evaluate maternal-infant behavior in the home setting. It may be used for children above 34 months of age, if necessary. Trained observers familiar with the infant's home behavior with the caregiver complete the set. The observer must indicate how similar or not similar an observed behavior is with reference to behaviors described in the Q-set. The set has undergone several validity studies and has demonstrated that it is helpful in identifying securely and insecurely attached infants under 1 year of age.

Measures of Play

Belsky and Most Free-Play Procedure

Belsky, J., & Most, R. (1981). From exploration to play: A cross sectional study of infant free-play behavior. *Developmental Psychology, 17,* 630.

The Free-Play Procedure was developed to identify and validate the developmental progression of infant play behaviors. It consists of a 30-minute home-based free-play observation with a set of standardized toys. The examiner and caregiver remain passive toward the child and simply observe the child's play behaviors. Observed play is classified into one of 12 forms that emerge in developmental sequence. These behaviors include mouthing, simple visually guided manipulation, functional manipulation, relational play, functional relational play, enactive naming, pretense behaviors, pretense behaviors directed toward others, substitution of objects and actions, sequence of single pretense acts, sequence of related but distinct pretense acts, and pretense play in which two objects are substituted. The 12 behaviors may be examined individually or grouped into three global ratings: low-level undifferentiated play, active transitional play, or high-level decontextualized pretense play. The scale has been demonstrated to accurately describe the developmental progression of play.

Morgan, Harmon, and Bennett Procedure (MMBP)

Morgan, G., Harmon, R., & Bennett, C. (1976). A system for coding and scoring infants' free play with objects. *Catalogue of Selected Documents in Psychology, 6,* 105.

The MMBP consists of a free-play observation of children 8 to 24 months of age in either the home or clinical setting. Free play with a standardized set of toys is observed for 40 minutes. The procedure is designed to distinguish exploratory play from cognitively mature play. Play is scored as representing one of six categories that are subsumed under three levels: passive exploration, active play, and high-level play. The observer records the specific toy used by the child, as well as mother-infant interactions during the play session. The instrument correlates nicely with scores obtained on the Bayley Scale, particularly for children under 1 year of age who score well on the scale.

Lowe and Costello Symbolic Play Test (SPT)

Lowe, M., & Costello, A. (1976). Manual for the Symbolic Play Test. Windsor, England: Nelson Publishing.

The SPT assesses infants 12 to 36 months of age. Infants are presented with four sets of standardized toys, one set at a time. The caregiver is present for the assessment but is asked not to elicit or engage the child with any particular toy. No time constraints are offered. Each toy set has a specific coding sequence/scheme whereby the frequency of specific play behaviors is recorded and percentages of play behaviors/levels are computed. Test results are used to monitor increasing sophistication and decentration in free play with increasing age.

McCune-Nicolich Procedure

McCune-Nicolich, L. (1983). A manual for analyzing free play. New Brunswick, NJ: Department of Educational Psychology, Rutgers University.

This procedure is designed to assess more complex symbolic play of older toddlers. The procedure employs a 30-minute observation of free play in the home setting with a standardized set of 36 toys designed to elicit symbolic free play. The mother and examiner are present but do not attempt to elicit free-play samples. The play behaviors that are assessed are categorized into simple presymbolic schemes or auto-symbolic schemes. The scale is based on the premise that play unfolds in a schematic, developmental progression that can be observed and measured/described. Time sampling is not used, unlike in many play behavior measures.

Belsky Procedure

Belsky, J., Garduque, L., & Hrncir, E. (1984). Assessing performance, competence, and executive capacity in infant play: Relations to home environment and security of attachment. *Developmental Psychology, 20,* 406.

This procedure involves a 10-minute observation of infant free play, followed by a period during which the examiner engages the child in more sophisticated play behaviors through the use of verbal prompts and modeling. Both the free-play and elicited play behaviors are coded and scored. Three different scores are derived: performance, competence, and executive capacity. The premise is that highly motivated children will be more likely to exhibit their full capacities during the free-play procedure and that elicitation will do little to boost play performance. It is implied, through this procedure, that individual differences in infant motivation are related not only to cognitive competence but also to social competence. Review of the procedure has validated the fact that both free and elicited play increase in complexity over time, although changes may not be predictive of attachment. It is further assumed that play not only reflects both social and cognitive competence but also may, at least in part, mediate the relationship between early social relations and later cognitive competence.

Fewell's Play Assessment Scale (PAS)

Fewell, R. (1986). *Play Assessment Scale* (5th revision). Unpublished manuscript. Seattle, WA: University of Washington.

The PAS examines perceptual and cognitive skills or processes of children 2 through 36 months old through observing the child's interactions with a series of toy sets designed to elicit a broad range of skills of progressive sophistication. Two conditions are built into the procedure. The first focuses on spontaneous play, and the second employs verbal cues and physical modeling. This allows the examiner the opportunity to view more sophisticated skills of the child. The PAS emphasizes the importance of the observer recording the success of specific verbal and physical prompts because this information is valuable to teachers and others interested in measuring and promoting the child's development.

Bromwich Play Assessment Checklist for Infants (PACFI)

Bromwich, R. (1981). *Play Assessment Checklist for Infants.* (Available from author, Department of Educational Psychology, School of Education, California State University).

The PACFI is designed as an observational aid for EI professionals. It uses a standardized toy set to tap cognitive functioning in spontaneous free-play settings among children 9 to 30 months old. It also includes procedures for assessing temperamental characteristics of the child. Further, it assesses social/linguistic behavior toward the parent/caregiver as well as cognitive/motivational behavior toward the play behavior. The emphasis is placed on the quality of the child's functioning with the premise that cognitive and affective development are inseparable in infancy. The information gained from this procedure is important for EIs in any attempts to provide developmentally supportive environments for intervention.

Assessment of Gesture, Pragmatics, Language Comprehension, and Language Expression

Significant overlap exists between assessment tools for the measurement of behaviors thought to reflect gesture, pragmatics, language comprehension, and language expression. Hence, the following assessment tools reflect instruments that assess each of these domains within the framework of a comprehensive assessment of infant/toddler communicative status.

Communication and Symbolic Behavior Scales

Weatherby, A., & Prizant, B. (1991). Communication and Symbolic Behavior Scales (CSBS). Chicago: Riverside Publishing.

The CSBS is a norm-referenced standardized assessment for identifying children who are at risk for communication delay and for establishing and monitoring changes in the child's communication, social-affective, and symbolic development. It is designed for children between 9 months and 6 years of age (functional communication age between 9 months and 2 years). The scale integrates both parent and professional observations on 22 items. Each item is rated on a 1- to 5-point scale. Scoring includes raw, scaled, cluster, percentile, rank, and standard scores. Determination of language stages, which include prelinguistic, one-word, late one-word, and multiword performance, are included. It also affords links to curriculum suggestions for intervention. It provides accurate focus on reciprocal communication, regardless of communication mode. Normative data on typical and atypical groups is provided.

MacArthur Communicative Development Inventories (CDI)

Fenson, P., Dale, P. S., Reznick, J. S., Thal, D., Bates, E., Hartung, J. P., Pethick, S., & Reilly, J. S. (1993). *MacArthur Communicative Development Inventories.* San Diego, CA: Singular Publishing Group.

The CDI is a comprehensive set of parent report instruments to assess communication development from 8 to 36 months of age. It has been previously demonstrated that parent report can be used effectively as an accurate picture of the child's language and communication development. The items are arranged into 22 categories in Part I. In Part II, 125 items pertaining to grammatical development are included. Some items ask about the frequency of use of various grammatical forms. Other items include a forced choice format in which the parent is asked to indicate which of two forms sounds most like what the child might use. In addition, the parent is asked to give examples of three of the child's longest sentences. The validity of the CDI has been demonstrated, as has the reliability of parent report as a means of data collection. It is helpful in providing an in-depth picture of the child's vocabulary by form or class or a detailed profile of his or her mastery of specific syntactic features. The CDI has not been widely used to identify children with delayed language or communication skills and is not as readily applicable for structuring an intervention program as a result.

Observation of Communicative Interaction (OCI)

Klein, M., & Briggs, M. (1987). Facilitating mother-infant communicative interaction in mothers of high-risk infants. *Journal of Childhood Communication Disorders, 4,* 91.

The OCI is a procedure that allows for the assessment of communicative interactions between mother and infant. The OCI was developed for use as an informal observation guide to assist EI staff in describing the interaction strategies used by parents while interacting with their infants. It is intended for use as a clinical observation tool and should be used as an informal guide to qualitative assessment of relative strengths and weakness of caregiver-infant interaction. It is not designed as a research tool. The data collected may be used to monitor change over time. It may be used to provide guidance in planning individual target goals, intervention strategies, and interaction activities. It is administered during an observation in which the caregiver is engaged in a routine interaction with the infant. It outlines 10 interaction categories around which observations are structured. It is structured to yield valuable information regarding the quality and style of mother-infant interaction.

The Language Development Survey (LDS): A Screening Tool for Delayed Language Toddlers

Rescorla, L. (1989). The language development survey: A screening tool for delayed language in toddlers. *Journal of Speech and Hearing Disorders, 2,* 587.

The LDS was designed as a quick and efficient screening tool for the identification of language delay in 2-year-old children. It consists of a one-page double-sided survey form with a checklist of about 300 vocabulary words arranged alphabetically by semantic category. The parent is asked to check off each word the child uses spontaneously. The parent is also asked whether or not the child uses word combinations and is asked to give three examples of the child's best sentences. The LDS has, over time, been shown to be an effective tool for the identification of toddlers who are slow to talk. The results of the LDS have been shown to correlate nicely with more structured standardized measures of vocabulary and cognitive performance. It is not of assistance in structuring intervention for children with communicative delay but can serve to identify only.

Rossetti Infant-Toddler Language Scale: A Measure of Communication and Interaction (ITLS)

Rossetti, L. (1990). *The Rossetti Infant-Toddler Language Scale: A measure of communication and interaction.* Moline, IL: LinguiSystems.

The ITLS is a criterion-referenced measure of communication skills for children birth through 36 months of age. It allows for the collection of responses through parental report, directly elicited behaviors, or spontaneously observed behaviors. It consists of seven communication domains, which include interaction, attachment, play, pragmatics, gesture, language comprehension, and language expression. In addition, it provides a comprehensive format for collecting valuable parental data in a case-history format. Scoring is simple and affords the examiner the option of moving beyond desired ceiling levels to identify emerging communication skills and specific areas of developmental progress. This is a valuable component because it assists the EI in structuring intervention activities that are suited to specific emerging communication behaviors demonstrated by the child. It is widely used and readily adaptable to the home or clinical setting.

Transdisciplinary Play-Based Assessment (TPBA)

Linder, T. (1990). *Transdisciplinary Play-Based Assessment: A functional approach to working with young children.* Baltimore: Paul H. Brookes.

The TPBA is a curriculum-embedded assessment tool for use with children from infancy to 6 years of age. It is suitable for arena use. It assesses cognitive, social-emotional, communication and language, and sensorimotor skills. It is designed to be used by professionals representing all EI disciplines. It is highly individualized, naturalistic, and assists with structuring a comprehensive intervention program. It provides team ideas of play behaviors, team assessment of play suggestions, and play-based curriculum planning sheets. It contains observation and summary worksheets that include more detailed subcategories of abilities in each developmental domain. Team members are able to identify child strengths, areas of concern, and areas of readiness. The results readily allow for the implementation of an intervention program.

AEPS Measurement for Birth to Three Years (AEPS)

Bricker, D. (1993). *AEPS measurement for birth to three years.* Baltimore: Paul H. Brookes.

The AEPS is a curriculum-based assessment/evaluation system that encourages natural learning opportunities for children in the developmental range of birth to 6 years of age. AEPS provides a framework for developing worthwhile, individualized goals and objectives. The first volume (birth to 3 years of age) allows for the functional measurement of skills in infants and children in six developmental domains: fine motor, gross motor, adaptive, cognitive, social-communication, and social. The AEPS is adaptable for children with special needs. Assessment is performed while the child is engaged in naturally occurring activities. The system does not generate age-equivalent scores, but rather identifies progress through the curriculum provided as part of the system. The third volume (3 to 6 years of age) is divided into the same sections as the first volume. There is a family interest survey included that consists of a 30-item checklist that helps to identify interests and priorities that may be addressed in the child's IEP/IFSP. Overall, this is a very effective tool for the identification of specific areas in which to focus intervention activities.

Clinical Linguistic and Auditory Milestone Scale (CLAMS)

Capute, A., Palmer, F., Shapiro, B., Wachtel, R., Schmidt, S., & Ross, A. (1986). A clinical linguistic and auditory milestone scale (CLAMS): Prediction of cognition in infancy. *Developmental Medicine and Child Neurology, 28,* 762.

The CLAMS is designed for use in assessing receptive and expressive language through direct observation and parental report. The CLAMS recognizes the reliability of parental report and uses parent-provided data as part of the assessment procedure. It is designed for use with children 1 to 36 months of age. It does not readily lend itself to structuring intervention but can be a helpful adjunct to more standardized assessment tools. It is easy to use regardless of assessment setting.

Receptive-Expressive Emergent Language Scale (REEL)

Bzoch, K., & League, R. (1971). Assessing language skills in infancy: A handbook for the multidimensional analysis of emergent language. Baltimore: University Park Press.

The purpose of the REEL is to identify young children who may have delays in communication that necessitate early intervention focusing on the communication domain. The REEL is administered primarily through a parent information interview. The scale allows for considerable license in probing for information on each item. Direct observation of reported behaviors is suggested but not mandatory. It is designed for use with children birth through 36 months of age. Six items are listed for each 1-month interval. Year 2 spans 2-month intervals. Six items are listed for each age span for both receptive and expressive language items.

Sequenced Inventory of Communication Development—Revised (SICD)

Hedrick, D., Prather, E., & Tobin, A. (1986). *Sequenced Inventory of Communication Development*. Seattle, WA: University of Washington Press.

The SICD attempts to assess systematically receptive and expressive communication development for children age 4 months to 4 years. The ultimate purpose is to increase efficiency for remedial programming both in the home and in the educational setting. There are two major sections to the inventory: an expressive and a receptive section. The expressive section is designed to represent a cross-section of linguistic and psychological paradigms. There are five domains represented on the scale: initiating, imitating, responding, verbal output, and articulation. Items represented on the scale include a developmental range from 4 to 48 months.

Preschool Language Scale (Revised)

Zimmerman, I., Steiner, V., & Pond, R. (1979). *Preschool Language Scale.* Columbus, OH: Charles Merrill.

The PLS was designed to detect language strengths and deficiencies. It consists of two main sections: auditory and verbal ability. A supplementary articulation section is also included. The auditory section consists of subtests that require a nonverbal response such as pointing. The verbal ability section consists of items that require the child to name or explain. The articulation section requires the child to say words and sentences after the examiner. The scale is designed for use with children between 18 months and 7 years of age.

Infant Scale of Communicative Intent (ICI)

Coplan, J. (1982). An assessment tool: The infant scale of communicative intent. *Update Pediatrics,* 7, 1.

The ICI is a nonstandardized, descriptive measure developed to meet the needs of a population of infants with developmental concerns. The scale was devised from published tests, research data, and clinical observations and experience. It emphasizes the child's intent to communicate in several modes and to interact socially with others. The scale consists of a checklist containing 10 behaviors at 1-month intervals from birth to 18 months of age. The items at each age are intended to provide a general description of the communicative behavior of children at each stage. The scale is administered by observation, direct testing, or parental report.

Assessing Prelinguistic and Early Linguistic Behaviors in Developmentally Young Children

Olswang, L., Stoel-Gammons, C., Coggins, T., & Carpenter, R. (1987). *Assessing prelinguistic and early linguistic behaviors in developmentally young children.* Seattle, WA: University of Washington Press.

This system consists of a manual for describing an assessment protocol for children functioning between 9 and 24 months of age. The program includes five scales assessing the following aspects of prelinguistic and early linguistic development: cognitive antecedents to word meaning, play, communicative intent, language comprehension, and language production.

CHAPTER
4

General Considerations for Communication-Based Intervention

❝ Language is the single best predictor of future cognition in a young child. Prelinguistic and language development occur in an orderly sequence. . . .studies are now demonstrating, however, a continuum from the prelinguistic skills of infancy to the language skills of the preschool years. ❞

(Capute, Palmer, Shapiro, 1987)

The concept of continuum of risk is important for the early interventionist to keep in mind. The principle behind this concept is that the beginning point for delayed communication skills is not at the moment the child fails to utter his or her first word at an age-appropriate phase in development. Rather, the child who does not demonstrate age-appropriate communication development does so due to factors that be may linked to influences relating to earlier events (environmental, biological, or both). Take, for example, the child who is born at 26 weeks' gestational age and with a birth weight of 1150 g. Further, assume that the child is born in a small rural hospital and immediately following birth is transported via helicopter to a large NICU several hundred miles from home. The mother may have a fleeting glimpse, at best, of her child before he is stabilized and transported. If she has other children at home, has transportation difficulties, or is a single parent, her opportunity to visit the child in the NICU is significantly compromised. Where does the continuum of risk begin for this child? It begins right away and continues to increase as the mother is not afforded opportunity to interact with the child, and the child has a host of medical risk factors attached to it. It becomes imperative that the EI adopt the view that risk for communication delay and the corollary risk for school failure begin early and that communication-based intervention must, likewise, begin as early as possible.

Lockwood (1994) has noted that children with early communication delay are at high risk for later developing learning problems once they reach school age. Lockwood further suggests that it is imperative that communication delay be detected early, because early detection is critical for academic and emotional health. A further benefit of early detection is that caregivers learn what they can do to help their child. In addition, caregivers, health care providers, early intervention personnel, and educators can recognize that a child is at risk for learning difficulties. Appropriate intervention can, therefore, begin early. Lockwood (1994) provides additional information about various risk factors present in children with communication delay that relate to increased risk for later school failure. Table 4–1 presents these risk factors in summary form.

The need for early identification of communication impairment is important if later school problems are to be avoided. Many early interventionists share a common frustrating experience noted when caregivers are asked when they first had any degree of concern regarding a child's communication development. Many caregivers will suggest that they initially became concerned when the child was quite young. If they are subsequently asked to whom they told their concerns, the usual response is no one or some professional (generally the physician, but not in every instance). The usual response such parents receive from various professionals is to suggest that they not worry, but rather wait and see what changes take place over time. Parents frequently express frustration at not having their concerns taken seriously. Clinicians, likewise, become frustrated when they learn that parental concern was expressed to appropriate professionals early in a child's life, but a referral for communication assessment and intervention was not made. When caregivers are asked why the person to whom they expressed initial concern did not suggest a communication-based assessment, the general response is that they were told that children do not learn to talk until approximately 1 year, thus assessment of communication skills and potential communication-based intervention cannot be provided for children under 12 months of age. *The entire early intervention team must challenge this notion.*

How should the EI respond when faced with objections to early communication assessment/intervention? One suggestion is to inquire whether the person resisting early referral sees the need for

TABLE 4–1 Risk Factors for Communication Disorders

Perinatal Infection
  Cytomegalovirus, rubella, herpes, syphilis, toxoplasmosis

Birth Weight
  Birth weight less than 1,500 g

Ototoxic Drugs
  If taken for a period of 10 days or longer

Deviations in Sucking or Feeding
  Considered positive if accompanied by a NICU stay, questionable if not accompanied by a NICU stay, positive if problems persist and are accompanied by a lag in early speech development

Birth Defects
  Cleft lip/palate, submucous cleft, bifid or missing uvula, pseudo clefting of the nose, micrognathia, morphological abnormalities of the pinna, auricular tags, dysmorphic appearance, hydrocephalus, proven chromosomal syndrome

Blood/Exchange Transfusion for Hyperbilirubinemia
  Hyperbilirubinemia, severe jaundice, kernicterus or premature liver present

Family History of Hearing Loss
  Hearing loss in family attributed to hereditary etiology

Family History of Speech Problems or Learning Disabilities
  Positive if present in child's immediate family or first-degree relative

Adapted from "Early Speech and Language Indicators for Later Learning Problems: Recognizing a Language Organization Disorder" by S. Lockwood, 1994, *Infants and Young Children, 7*, p. 43.

referral to the physical or occupational therapist before the child reaches 1 year of age. The general response is that referral to the occupational or physical therapist is readily made. The EI interested in promoting early referral for communication assessment and intervention should then ask why the referral is made to the occupational and physical therapist if children do not walk until approximately 1 year of age. The usual response is that a variety of developmental achievements must take place before the child is able to walk. In other words, there is an assortment of precursors to walking. The point to be made is readily apparent. There are numerous precursors to communication development. In reviewing the developmental follow-up data presented in Chapter 1, it is quite apparent that communication skills are the single developmental domain that consistently separates no-risk from at-risk children. Further, communication skills are highly correlated with school success. Those children entering school with deficits in communication skills generally struggle in the early elementary grades. This pattern of early struggle can prove difficult to break from. So, it is imperative that particular attention be directed to communication development from the earliest ages. It simply makes no sense to refer to other early intervention professionals and exclude the communication specialist.

Although it might appear that the previous discussion is suggesting that one discipline represented on the early intervention team should be preferred over another, nothing could be further from the truth. In essence, the point to be made is that at-risk children, regardless of the specifics of their risk status, display communication delay more frequently than any other developmental deficit. And if communication skills are the single best predictor of future cognition and subsequent school performance, it becomes compulsory that care be directed toward early assessment and intervention for potential communication delay. The entire EI team, including the medical community, must be made aware of this principle.

The concept of continuum of risk, likewise, has significant implications regarding what information is communicated to caregivers at the outset of their concern for the development of their child. For example, what information is communicated to parents on the day their child is dismissed from the neonatal intensive care nursery? Parents are generally relieved that they are finally permitted to take their child home. Is adequate information shared with them about the continuum of risk that the child presents relative to the potential for later communication delay and potential school difficulties? In many instances, information of this nature is not effectively communicated to parents. The result is that they may not be as vigilant as possible in checking communication development. Although no EI can pinpoint with certainty which children will display communication delay or the degree of delay, if present, at the very least caregivers should be informed of any potential for delay and alerted to the availability of assessment and intervention services. Information provided to physicians (Largo, Molinari, Pinto, & Weber, 1986) suggests that the physician should expect at least a minor delay in communication development in preterm children. With the linkage between communication delay and school performance as previously specified, the physician should at least be aware of the added risk. Is information of this nature adequately provided to parents? In many instances, the answer is no and age of identification of communication delay is postponed, thus directly reducing the efficacy of treatment.

One facet of the communication EIs have with parents relates to school readiness. Parents should be informed that their child is at risk for communication delay and that the overall long-range goal is that their child be as ready for school as possible when the child reaches school age. Information of this nature provides parents with a greater understanding of continuum of risk. As a result, they do not falsely assume that once a child returns home from the intensive care nursery, vigilance relative to the child's development can be reduced. This simply is not the case. Yet, lack of such vigilance is one reason why early referral does not take place as it should.

The information to follow is designed to alert the EI to a host of general issues about early communication-based intervention. This chapter provides the EI with a variety of suggestions regarding communication-based intervention for children from birth through 2 years of age. The appendix at the end of this chapter lists materials for communication-based intervention.

MODELS OF SERVICE DELIVERY

Conditions unique to each community dictate, in large measure, the basic setting in which communication-based early intervention services are provided. There are variations in intensity of intervention, duration of services, personnel involved, and the specific setting in which services are delivered. In addition, variations relative to each family served may likewise influence the type and setting of intervention services. One traditional manner of grouping models of service delivery is by the type of setting in which the infant-toddler receives services. Although not exclusive, one paradigm of service delivery includes services delivered in a center (center-based services), services delivered primarily in the home setting, and combination home-center service delivery models. Table 4–2 displays various characteristics of each of these service delivery approaches. The information that follows contains material about each setting in which communication-based early intervention services may be delivered.

McWilliam and Strain (1993) suggest that various principles regarding early intervention services should be followed, regardless of whether the intervention services are delivered in a center, in the home, or in a home-center combination. These principles, as outlined by McWilliam and Strain, include the following:

1. Whatever the service delivery model, it should be the least restrictive and most natural environment for the child and family.

2. All services should be family centered and responsive to families' priorities.

TABLE 4–2 Early Intervention Service Delivery Options

Center-Based Programs

Group activities provide consultation and training for parents and intervention services for the child.

Child may spend the day (or part of the day) in a developmentally appropriate classroom. This may include time with typically developing peers.

There are specialized classrooms and interventions to serve only children with developmental needs.

Skilled nursing care in a group setting is available for children with complex health needs or children dependent on technology.

Home-Based Programs

A range of supports is available, including materials, information, advice, instruction, and emotional support.

In-home parent support and/or parent training is available and may include direct intervention with the child.

Child-care provider receives support and training to include the child with special needs.

Home-Center Combinations

Programs are combined, including center-based child programs and home-visiting components.

Adapted from "Models of Service Delivery" (p. 184), by D. Bryant and M. Graham in *Implementing Early Intervention*, edited by D. Bryant and M. Graham, 1993, New York: Guilford Press.

3. The services that are provided should be delivered in a transdisciplinary fashion. This allows maximal child and family participation.

4. Service delivery practices should be predicated on empirical results and family values.

5. The services received by a child and family should be individualized and developmentally appropriate.

Center-Based Early Intervention Services

A center-based early intervention model implies that all intervention activities are provided in the context of an early intervention center. Centers of this nature may be affiliated with a hospital, the local schools, private rehabilitation agencies, county-based child development centers, or local service providers that furnish an array of intervention activities in a central location. In many instances, center-based services are provided for children who were identified early and who received their initial early intervention services (following hospital discharge) in the home. Following a period of home-based services, the child and family usually transition to a center-based service delivery system. There are various benefits of center-based services. The specific environments in which center-based services are provided are as varied as the professionals working with infants and toddlers. Filler (1983) lists several benefits of center-based services. First, parents and children have greater access to staff and a variety of services. One strength of center-based EI services is that additional professional expertise is readily available, whereas in the home setting one primary early intervention provider is present. Second, parents have greater opportunity to interact with other parents of children with special needs. The benefits of interaction of this type should not be underestimated. It is important that parents of special needs children realize that they are not alone in the frustrations they experience. Parents find it quite supportive to have another set of parents with whom they might share their problems. A final benefit to center-based intervention is the availability of other services. Should any specialized services be needed, they are more readily available to the child and family.

Within the center-based model of early intervention, a variety of options are available. Table 4–3 presents several center-based types. As may be readily observed, changes in the traditional center-based setting have taken place over the past 15 years. The options described in Table 4–3 provide services that vary in intensity, professionals involved, access to typically developing children, and caregiver involvement. The specific routines employed in various center-based settings are characterized by significant curricular diversity, as well as diversity in physical setup and types of professionals involved. However, regardless of the specific setting in which center-based early intervention activities are provided, heavy emphasis on communication skills is paramount.

With the exception of early intervention services provided in the intensive care nursery, center-based settings have been in existence (although not primarily geared toward children from birth to 3 years of age) for some time. Services provided in the context of the intensive care nursery represent the most recent application of the concept of early intervention (developmentally appropriate care). The discussion that follows is intended to acquaint the EI with a broad array of issues related to developmentally appropriate care in the framework of the NICU. The implications for enhancing overall communication skills are apparent.

TABLE 4–3   Center-Based Early Intervention Options

Parent Child Centers

   Group activities are designed to provide consultation and training for parents and intervention for the child.

Developmental Child Care

   The child spends part of the day in a developmentally appropriate setting/classroom in a community-based setting, perhaps with typically developing children included.

Reverse Mainstreaming

   The child receives services in a specialized early intervention classroom that includes some children without special needs.

Traditional Specialized Intervention

   Classrooms are designed to provide specialized instruction and intervention geared only for children with special needs.

Medical Child Care Settings

   Children with specialized health needs receive intervention services in a skilled nursing setting with children displaying similar health concerns.

Adapted from "Models of Service Delivery" (p. 184), by D. Bryant and M. Graham in *Implementing Early Intervention*, edited by D. Bryant and M. Graham, 1993, New York: Guilford Press.

NICU-Based Intervention

Competencies Needed to Provide NICU Early Intervention

A question asked frequently by early intervention professionals relates to their desire to provide developmentally appropriate care in the context of the intensive care nursery: "I am a (fill in the specific discipline) and I would like to gain access to the intensive care nursery to provide developmental intervention. How do I gain such access?" A second question, closely related to the first, is this: "I am a (fill in the specific discipline) with access to the NICU. What in the world do I do?" Both of these questions demonstrate the increased desire of EIs to facilitate optimal developmental performance for NICU graduates. The motivation behind each of these questions is also apparent for those clinicians that provide services outside of the hospital setting. Many school districts, community agencies, and other service delivery settings provide intervention services for children from birth.

   Modern advances in acute neonatal care have resulted in dramatically improved survival rates for low-birth-weight infants and older children with major congenital abnormalities. Medical techniques and practice have lowered the mortality rate significantly for many children that would not have survived even 5 years ago. One by-product of significantly lowered mortality is that the medical community is now asking a new question. Although attention will never be directed away from issues related to improved survival, in the present climate of improved survival the questing has shifted to the manner in which care is provided and how developmental outcome may be enhanced. In other words, the question is no longer primarily "Can we save more babies?" but rather, "Can we improve developmental outcome for survivors?" This improved survival rate has resulted, however, in an increase in the number of young children with chronic health conditions that may affect on developmental skill mastery. These children often undergo long periods of hospitalization following birth or require frequent rehospitalization during the first years of life. In recent years considerable attention has been focused on provision of developmental intervention for infants in the NICU or infants in pediatric intensive care units (PICUs).

Although a significant amount of attention has been recently directed toward developmental care in these settings, few professionals received adequate training during undergraduate and graduate education. Where are the appropriate skills learned? How does the EI gain the needed base of information and appropriate clinical experience? What is the basic knowledge base for effective developmental care? The answer to these questions is quite important if effective developmental intervention in these settings is to become a reality. The EI who functions in the NICU must fill a variety of roles if effective services are to be delivered. These roles include the following (Katz, Pokorni, & Long, 1989):

- *Infant specialist:* In fulfilling this role, the EI must become intimately acquainted with the physical and behavioral responses that critically ill infants display. In addition, the EI needs information and skills in intervention strategies with both the ill full-term infant as well as the infant who is premature. Behavioral responses and intervention strategies differ for infants at different stages of development. The EI must be prepared to work with infants at each of these stages.
- *Facilitator and consultant:* Effective service provision in the NICU requires that the EI function as a facilitator and consultant with skills to observe, understand, and communicate about the infant's behavioral responses to the environment. This role suggests that the EI may best intervene on the part

of the infant not through direct hands-on services to the infant, but rather through timely suggestions to the parents and the staff. This role suggests that the EI who is able to interact with adults and work with infants at the same time will be effective in the services provided.

- *Parent/caregiver educator:* The EI working in the NICU will also function as a parent educator. In this role, the EI assists the parents in understanding their infant's sometimes unexpected and immature behavioral responses. The EI may also assist the parents in noticing the infant's communicative cues and in developing appropriate responses to these cues.
- *Program developer and advocate:* In this capacity the EI will need to keep abreast of current research findings and work to apply these advances to develop more appropriate intervention strategies. Ongoing advocacy may be needed in the NICU to ensure that "best practice" is always applied in the NICU for developmentally appropriate care. Historically, NICUs have been concerned primarily with effective medical intervention. Now, equal emphasis is directed toward making the NICU experience as least noxious for the infant as possible. Although recognizing the critical need for ongoing and often noxious medical treatment, the EI will need to advocate for the ongoing developmental needs of both the infant and the parents.

VandenBerg (1993) provides additional information designed to address questions about competencies needed to work in the NICU. VandenBerg notes that the developmental specialist may represent any one of several academic disciplines, including occupational, speech, or physical therapy; education; social work; psychology; medicine; or nursing. However, regardless of primary academic discipline, a basic educational and clinical background is needed to implement effective developmental care. The knowledge base described by VandenBerg covers both primary and specialized knowledge.

PRIMARY KNOWLEDGE BASE. The primary knowledge base needed to implement developmental care in the NICU is in three basic areas. The first of these is knowledge of typical infant development. This includes familiarity with theory and research in normal infant development during prenatal and perinatal stages of maturation. It should include information about how infants interact with their environment and how social and environmental matters affect the child. The second area of basic knowledge includes information on atypical infant development. Risk factors regarding prenatal and perinatal development should be fully understood by the EI. This includes information relating to disabilities and disabling conditions and their effect on families. The final area of primary knowledge described by VandenBerg includes theory and research about family systems and knowledge of attachment theory and parent-infant interactions (as well as factors that enhance risk for parent interaction difficulties). This includes a broad base of knowledge about how to better meet family needs, assess family needs effectively, and enhance the likelihood that effective professional-parent relationships develop.

SPECIALIZED KNOWLEDGE. Specialized knowledge relating to developmental care falls into seven main categories as described by VandenBerg (1993).

1. *Knowledge of fetal and newborn brain development:* This includes familiarity with the function of specific areas of the brain, sensory impact on brain development, principles of brain plasticity, as well as other specific and unique characteristics of the premature infant's brain and its functions following birth.

2. *Knowledge of medical conditions to which premature and full-term neonates are susceptible:* Chapter 1 in this text provides an overview of the most frequently occurring conditions in premature infants.

3. *Knowledge of how specific medical conditions affect the normal development and the developmental sequelae of various conditions:* This includes specific illnesses, medical equipment and drugs used in the nursery, and specific medical treatments and procedures.

4. *Knowledge of neonatal preterm and full-term infant behaviors and development:* This includes cognizance of sensory development, including vision, auditory, tactile, and vestibular function. It also includes awareness of motor system functioning (posture, tone, and movement patterns), sleep-wake cycles, state development, and infant behaviors of stress and stability.

5. *Knowledge of the environment of the nursery:* The EI needs a basic understanding of the nature of the nursery (noise, touch, lighting, temperature, miscellaneous interventions, and handling) and how these issues affect an infant's development during periods of illness.

6. *Knowledge of staffing patterns and routines and the cultural patterns present in each NICU:* This area of knowledge includes all issues relating to general caregiving while the child is hospitalized.

7. *Knowledge of information concerned with parenting in the NICU:* This includes parental perceptions of the NICU, parental reactions to having an ill child, and the general emotional issues faced by parents. This may include helping parents deal with medical emergencies and the potential that their child may die.

In addition to these areas of primary specialized knowledge, VandenBerg (1993) describes a variety of issues related to supervised experience needed by the EI working in the NICU. These are presented in summary form in Table 4–4.

In addition to the areas of knowledge and supervised experience specified previously, other competencies needed for early intervention personnel are specified by Hanson and Brekken (1991). Although the issues identified by Hanson and Brekken are not directly specific to those EIs providing developmentally appropriate care in the NICU, the basic suggestions provided are fully applicable to NICU personnel. The suggestions provided by Hanson and Brekken include competencies in assessment, development, and implementation of individualized intervention plans; professional interaction skills; and personal interaction skills. Assessment competencies include familiarity with assessment practices appropriate for each infant, the selection and utilization of appropriate assessment tools, and the ability to accurately interpret and report assessment results. For the EI to develop and implement an appropriate intervention program, there must be familiarity with a range of intervention options. In addition, the EI must be able to evaluate intervention programs for overall effectiveness. Finally, the EI must possess professional and personal interaction skills for effective functioning. This includes the ability to work collaboratively with families and team members. Table 4–5 identifies characteristics recognized by Hanson and Brekken that apply to all early intervention personnel, regardless of employment setting or primary population. Fenichel and Eggbeer (1991) provide additional suggestions for preparing practitioners to work with infants, toddlers, and their families. These issues are applicable for EI personnel from various disciplines and without respect to primary place of employment or intervention setting.

Dunn, van Kleek, and Rossetti (1993) conducted a survey designed to assess the degree to which speech-language pathologists are trained to provide developmental care in the intensive care nursery. The

TABLE 4–4   Suggested Clinical Experiences for Developmental Enhancement in the NICU

Observations during the First 6 Months:
- Operation of NICU during all three shifts
- Rounds, staff conferences, NICU policy meetings
- Transport, admission, and discharge process
- Caregiving and treatment procedures, including positioning, handling, holding, suctioning, reintubating, placing lines, feeding, and respiratory care
- The entire range of neonatal states in response to handling and treatment procedures, including identification of what constitutes stress and what constitutes stability and coping strategies
- The entire range of neonatal behaviors in response to handling and treatment procedures
- Tracking a variety of NICU patients from admission to discharge, noting typical behaviors, setbacks, and progress

Learning during the Second 6 Months Should Include How To:
- Modify light, noise, and activity levels as appropriate for each infant
- Read infant signals appropriately and accurately
- Position infants
- Facilitate organized sleep and awake states
- Prevent and manage agitation and provide soothing strategies
- Facilitate and prepare for all levels of feeding, including oral nippling
- Facilitate parent's collaborative role of caring for infant at bedside with the medical staff
- Provide support to parents in understanding infant behavior and developmental needs

Adapted from "Basic Competencies to Begin Developmental Care in the Intensive Care Nursery," by K. VandenBerg, 1993, *Infants and Young Children, 6*, p. 52.

results demonstrate that although speech-language pathology, as a single discipline, has begun to establish a multifaceted role in the NICU setting, preservice preparation during undergraduate and graduate training is lacking. Twenty-six percent of the respondents in the survey currently working in a NICU received no training with the birth-to-3 population prior to graduation (not even units within a course). The majority (77%) had received no training dealing with the NICU population during their graduate training. Most speech-language pathologists obtained NICU training after graduation through various means: self-taught (82%) by reading journals, books, and assessment and intervention procedures; workshops (80%); and on-

TABLE 4-5   Personal Characteristics of All Early Intervention Personnel

- Enjoyment and appreciation of infants and toddlers
- Gentle, nurturing, and accepting style
- Collaborative attitude
- Optimistic, yet realistic, attitude and expectations for families, colleagues, and oneself
- Flexibility and sensitivity to changing conditions
- Openness to diversity in lifestyle, culture, religious belief, and language
- Self-awareness related to personal mental health, issues of codependence, and personal strengths and weaknesses
- Positive attitude and belief in families' abilities to identify and meet their own and their infants' or toddlers' needs with support
- Self-control and stressful situations handled calmly
- Sense of humor maintained

Adapted from "Early Intervention Personnel Model and Standards: An Interdisciplinary Field-Developed Approach," by M. Hanson and L. Brekken, 1991, *Infants and Young Children, 4*, p. 54.

the-job training (82%). The respondents described a variety of resources as being helpful in their overall training. The most frequently identified source of help was that received from other professionals providing services in the NICU. These professionals included occupational and physical therapists, child-infant specialists, nurses, neonatologists, clinical dieticians, and other speech-language pathologists. Seventy-five percent of the respondents believed that significant changes in graduate preparation should take place. Table 4–6 identifies the areas in which the respondents felt additional training was needed.

Rowan, Thorp, and McCollum (1990) describe an interdisciplinary practicum designed to foster infant-family and teaming competencies in speech-language pathologists. The design outlined by the authors is not directed specifically for those working in the NICU. However, it does present a helpful philosophy that can be incorporated into any training program designed to enhance service provision in the NICU. Table 4–7 summarizes the basic philosophy of the Rowan et al. program.

NICU Service Delivery

The EI concerned with providing developmentally appropriate care for infants in the NICU soon realizes that basically three avenues for

TABLE 4-6 Areas in Which the Professional Knowledge
Base Should Be Expanded

- Neonatal neuroanatomy and physiology
- Fetal development
- Normal and abnormal infant development in the following areas:
  Cognition
  Communication
  Feeding and oral motor skills
  Motor development
  Social-emotional development
- Positioning and handling of neonates
- Medical issues, terminology, diagnoses
- Medical equipment
- How associated problems affect the following:
  Developmental expectations
  Anatomy and physiology of the neonate
  Respiration

Adapted from "Current Roles and Continuing Needs of Speech-Language
Pathologists Working in Neonatal Intensive Care Units," by S. Dunn, A. van
Kleek, and L. Rossetti, 1993, *American Journal of Speech-Language
Pathology, 5*, p. 52.

service delivery exist. Services may be delivered directly to the child,
to the staff working in the NICU, or to the caregivers. There is significant overlap in this provision of services to the child, parents, or NICU
staff. Table 4–8 lists a variety of avenues for NICU service delivery.
The EI working in the NICU must be familiar with each of these proposed avenues of service provision. If the EI assumes that any one
avenue of services will justify entrance into the nursery, or maintain
service delivery, a significant mistake will be made. It is imperative
that the NICU-based EI understand the varied nature of the setting
and be prepared to deliver services to any of three constituencies identified here.

General NICU-Based Goals

Any discussion of NICU-based intervention should emphasize an
overview of general service provision goals in such a setting. Although
several disciplines may be involved in developmentally appropriate
care in the NICU, common goals are shared. In a discussion of intervention in the NICU, Hayes and Ensher (1994) provide an overview of

TABLE 4–7 Basic Philosophy of Interdisciplinary Training

Philosophy Related to Families

Parents are resourceful. The goal is to support parents in providing developmentally appropriate activities for their children, responding to family strengths, and building on their own natural interaction styles.

Philosophy Related to Children

Activities used in parent-infant play are based on developmentally appropriate, pleasurable parent-infant play that blends individual objectives for child growth into child-directed play that is supported and facilitated by the parents.

Philosophy Related to Teaming

A transdisciplinary approach to intervention is the goal. The approach implies that each of the team members involved will retain his or her own disciplinary expertise while benefiting from the knowledge and experience of the other disciplines. Group interactions are characterized by a spirit of collaboration in which team members operate interchangeably in the intervention process but continue to function as resources to one another in relation to their own disciplinary expertise.

Philosophy Related to Student Learning

Students preparing for careers as early interventionists for infants with disabilities and their families will develop skills and knowledge unique to their own disciplines in relation to the populations served, as well as skills and knowledge needed by any and all disciplines working with this population.

Adapted from "An Interdisciplinary Practicum to Foster Infant-Family and Teaming Competencies in Speech-Language Pathologists," by L. Rowan, E. Thorpe, and J. McCollum, 1990, *Infants and Young Children, 2,* p. 58.

intervention goals. The desire to address developmental, psychosocial, and family concerns leads to the suggestion that two primary goals exist for intervention in the NICU. The first of these is to reduce adverse and potentially detrimental stimuli to the lowest possible level. This relates, at least in part, to creating an optimally favorable nursery environment. This includes both the physical and social environment of the nursery. More details for meeting this goal are provided later in this chapter. The second general goal is to create supportive and developmentally appropriate environments for both newborns and their families. The general premise of these goals is that the concept of "risk" not only applies to the child's chances for survival, but that, as a result of life-threatening conditions, the infant has also experienced physiological and environmental circumstances that could potentially interfere with normal development. As a result, environ-

TABLE 4–8   Sample NICU-Based Developmental Intervention Activities

Services Directed Primarily toward the Infant
- Oral/motor feeding
- Infant neurodevelopmental assessment
- Positioning
- Calming
- Regulation of state
- Socio-communicative interaction
- Nutritional issues
- Handling
- Visual stimulation
- Auditory stimulation
- Tactile stimulation
- Vestibular-kinesthetic stimulation
- Physical/occupational/speech therapy

Services Directed Primarily toward the Staff
- Awareness of environment (noise, touch, light, procedures)
- Potential developmental sequelae
- Infant cues/signals
- Infant states while in the NICU
- Transition from state to state
- Infant self-regulatory styles
- Efficacy of developmentally appropriate care
- New advances in developmentally appropriate care
- Services offered by other disciplines
- Social environment of the NICU

Services Directed Primarily toward the Parents
- Explain roles of all persons working in the NICU
- Source of information relative to the NICU
- Assist with discharge planning and transition home
- Alert them to community services (if needed)
- Provide support during times of fear
- Assist in involving parents in caregiving while infant is hospitalized (put them to work)
- Put them in touch with other needed services/professionals
- Help them deal with infants' rapidly changing condition
- Assist them in struggles with bonding/attachment
- Answer questions about child's long-term development
- Help them deal with fears about child's long-term development
- Reinforce the need for developmental follow-up

mental, psychosocial, and family concerns must be addressed. Hayes and Ensher (1994) further note that three broad objectives relate to achieving the previously specified goals. These goals are directly related to the avenues of potential service provision specified elsewhere in this section.

The first objective is to educate the nursery staff (everyone working in the NICU) and the parents about the unique set of circumstances that ill infants face from the illness and the environment of the NICU. The entire NICU staff needs to be aware of and have knowledge of the types of stimulation (or protection) that can reduce problems caused by the NICU environment. Parents must learn about their babies and the manner in which the environment affects development. They must be shown how to identify and interpret the unique signals that their child sends. These include signs of stress, avoidance, or engagement cues distinctive to their child. Parents can be encouraged to touch, hold, and care for their infant as much as possible during the course of hospitalization. These activities enhance attachment and the parent's feeling of "ownership" of the child.

The second general objective for developing more appropriate nursery environments involves monitoring and assessing infant states. An understanding of premature infant states, as discussed in an earlier chapter, is essential for all working in the nursery. Lack of familiarity with issues related to attention, tuning out, in-turning, regulation of behavioral state, neurobehavioral response patterns, and feeding places the EI at a distinct disadvantage in structuring effective developmental care in the NICU. Lack of familiarity with infant states causes many parents to feel that their baby does not know that they (the parents) are there. Once parents question their value and participation in NICU activities, the seeds for attachment difficulties are sown.

The final objective for NICU-based intervention relates to enhancing the child's and parents' transition to the home setting. Planning for discharge and the family's transition should begin early during the child's hospital stay. Initial attention will have been directed toward the general medical condition of the child, which is a natural occurrence. However, the point is reached when emphasis must be directed toward how the child and parents will adjust once the child is dismissed from the NICU. This is a tenuous time—one filled with potential for either successful or difficult adjustments for the child and parents. Essential to this transition is basic training for the parents about home-care needs unique to their child, as well as postdischarge programs designed to assist parents with ongoing issues of care and development.

After long weeks or months of a child's hospitalization, parents are expected to take the child home and treat him or her like a "normal" child ("go home and be happy"). Yet, their experience has been anything but "normal." It is imperative that all EIs have a realistic view of the issues parents face when their child is discharged to the home setting. Barker (1991) provides some insight into the problems faced by parents on discharge. In Barker's investigation, several themes emerged following careful questioning of caregivers. The interviews with parents focused on parental expectations, concerns, general feelings, and the overall characteristics of the transition period. The themes that emerged are as follows:

1. *Ambivalence prior to discharge:* This is characterized by simultaneous feelings of desiring the child's discharge, while at the same time wanting the youngster to remain under the care of the professionals.

2. *The infant's impact on the family:* Parents express uncertainty about the amount of adjustment needed on the part of the entire family and how the child would be incorporated into the family following transition home.

3. *Issues of parental competence:* Parents express doubt about their ability to provide ongoing care for their infant and in their ability to recognize and manage problems that may arise at home.

4. *Infant vulnerability:* Parents express fear of illness, apnea, and the potential for the child's death while in the care of the parents.

5. *Feeding issues:* Mothers report concern about a lack of success with breastfeeding and significant difficulty with feeding, in general.

6. *Pervasiveness of the impact of prematurity:* Caregivers express an ongoing concern about the unexpected, as a factor of prematurity.

Barker concludes by noting that the transition home for parents and infants poses a unique set of concerns. She further notes that the entire EI team should be familiar with these and other issues to make the transition home as seamless and uneventful as possible.

A format for maintaining contact with families after discharge is essential. Several investigators have demonstrated improved child outcome in the presence of postdischarge programs (Gennaro, Brooten, & Bakewell-Sachs, 1991).

Environment of the Neonatal Intensive Care Nursery

A variety of suggestions designed to alter the nature of the NICU environment and nursery routine, thereby reducing stressors, can be made. Various aspects of the nature of the NICU environment and caregiving methods will be discussed in the material to follow.

LIGHTING. One significant environmental factor that must be taken into consideration in any discussion of reducing stressors in the NICU is lighting. Until recently, most infants in the NICU were exposed to relatively high levels of fluorescent light, often on a 24-hour basis (Peabody & Lewis, 1985). As a result, a significant degree of concern has been expressed about the possible detrimental effects on infants from exposure to high-intensity light. High-level lighting may contribute not only to stress the infant feels in the NICU but also to a higher incidence of significant eye disease in surviving infants. In one controlled study, a group of premature infants exposed to a high-level of lighting was compared to a matched group of infants for whom light levels were reduced. The results of this investigation had infants exposed to bright lights with a 30% greater incidence of retinopathy of prematurity (ROP) within a subgroup of infants weighing less than 1,000 g and a higher likelihood for ROP to occur throughout that sample (Glass et al., 1985). Information such as this has prompted many NICUs to pay particular attention to lighting and how alterations in lighting patterns may be introduced. What has emerged from this increased understanding of the effects of lighting is a movement toward flexibility in lighting patterns. These changes include reduction of lighting, allowing for periods of darkness, the use of indirect lighting, protecting infants from direct sunlight, lighting approximated to mirror wake-sleep cycles, and covering of incubators with blankets and diapers to shield children from excessive light (Catlett & Davis, 1990; Peabody & Lewis, 1985; Wolke, 1987). Most NICUs in the United States are currently making efforts to reduce environmental stress from light. Strategies designed to reduce harm from bright lighting in the NICU are summarized in Table 4–9. Further, increased attention is being directed toward color schemes in the nursery. For example, a very busy color scheme (one with child-friendly drawings on the walls) may increase the degree of agitation seen in many infants (particularly drug-exposed infants).

NOISE. Noise levels in the intensive care nursery are significantly higher than those in a typical newborn nursery and are also higher and of a different quality than those in the average home setting. Catlett

TABLE 4–9   Strategies for Reducing Bright Lighting in the NICU

● Cover the isolettes with blankets to reduce the amount of bright light that filters to individual isolettes.

● Dim the lights on a regular schedule, especially in transitional units, to reduce light levels as well as to promote normal day-night cycles.

● Cover the infant's eyes with patches during procedures employing heat and bilirubin lamps and shield infants in nearby isolettes.

Adapted from *Chronically ill and at-risk infants: Family Centered Intervention from Hospital to Home* (p. 249), by K. Katz, J. Pokorni, and T. Long, 1989, Palo Alto, CA: Vort Corporation.

and Davis (1990) have noted that noise levels in the NICU have been a major source of environmental stress for preterm infants. Schultz (1987) suggests that high-risk newborns have a much higher incidence of moderate to profound hearing loss (2.5% to 5%) than infants in the general population (1%). Long, Lucey, and Philip (1980) provided information on noise levels in a NICU over an 8-hour period. The overall results of their investigation revealed that the nursery staff contributed significantly to noise levels and that means for reducing environmental stress from noise are readily available. The effect of noise on the infant is further described in an investigation conducted by Catlett and Davis (1990). They reported that during a 2-hour observation in a NICU, 27 state changes were observed in five infants in response to loud noise. Additional observations of infant behavior in the Catlett and Davis study revealed that physiological distress was noted more than 75% of the time. This distress included heart rate increase and one episode of bradycardia resulting in the need for mechanical ventilation.

Another noise-related source of stress are the machines used in the NICU. These include phones, monitors, computers, printers, portable respiratory equipment, and the flow of people in and out of the NICU. Gottfried (1985) reported that the mean sound level in one NICU was 77 dB, and at times reached a peak intensity level of 109 dB. Children placed in an incubator experience a somewhat different noise environment than those in an open bassinet. Gottfried further noted that low-frequency sounds tend to penetrate the walls of incubators. Because human speech is in the higher frequency range, speech stimuli is often masked, to varying degrees, for the infant resting in an enclosed incubator. There is some controversy about whether noise levels in the NICU lead to permanent hearing loss in infants. One obvious result of the array of auditory stimuli to which infants are exposed while in the

NICU is the increased potential that the child is not able to readily
associate a noise it hears with the source of the noise. Hence, hospitalized babies may be less able to associate a particular voice with a particular face (Wolke, 1987). Table 4–10 outlines several strategies
designed to reduce the negative impact of loud noise on hospitalized
infants. What should be noted about these suggestions is that they are
simple to implement and should not cause a major disruption of routine for any NICU staff.

TOUCHING AND HANDLING. Touching and handling of infants during
hospitalization has been of increasing interest to NICU personnel for
a number of reasons. Does too much touch or inappropriate touch
contribute to the overall stress related to other factors in the nursery?
It is obvious that for medical intervention to be provided, some
degree of touch is necessary. What has emerged over the past 30 years
is not primarily related to the amount of touch, although it is readily
acknowledged that too much touch is inappropriate, but to a discussion of the type of touch. A variety of changes have taken place relative to touch.

Standard practice about caregiver access to infants in intensive
care, as well as issues related to touch, has changed dramatically. What
has materialized represents an evolution from a period when it was
thought best to keep ill infants in relative isolation, through a period
when very aggressive management was the norm for all premature or
ill infants, to the present discussion that relates not so much to the

TABLE 4–10 Strategies for Reducing Excess Noise in the NICU

- Gently lower the infant's head on the isolette mattress tray.
- Close portholes and isolette cabinets quietly.
- Set feeding bottles in places other than on top of isolettes.
- Eliminate finger tapping on isolettes.
- Move loud machinery (computer printers) out of the NICU.
- Encourage staff to silence alarms as soon as possible and to turn off the ventilator alarm prior to suctioning.
- Discontinue audible heart rate monitor beeps.
- Reduce talking over isolettes or across the room.
- Eliminate radios or reduce usage to designated periods, confining music to calm, soothing music.

Adapted from: *Chronically ill and at-risk infants: Family Centered Intervention from Hospital to Home* (p. 249), by K. Katz, J. Pokorni, and T. Long, 1989, Palo Alto, CA: Vort Corporation.

amount of touch but rather to the quality and type of touch. A 1942 report by Gleich listed the following "don'ts" concerning premature infants:

1. Don't handle the infant unnecessarily.

2. Don't allow anyone except the nurse and physician into the premature infant's room. Friends and relatives should be kept out.

3. Don't feed the premature infant more often than every three hours.

4. Don't allow the premature infant to sleep in a room with other children. Premature infants contract disease easily (p. 60).

It is relatively clear that what was considered "best practice" in 1942 included a climate in which the infant was allowed minimal contact with the world, minimal interactional opportunities, restricted chances for exposure to caretakers, and reduced experience with touch.

As the medical specialty of neonatology and corresponding expansion of the use of technology and drugs took place, the attitude shifted away from keeping the premature infant in a climate of isolation to one in which the full array of medical, technological, and pharmacological capabilities was applied to each infant in the NICU. In other words, the full brunt of medical capability was brought to bear for each infant. Hence, touch became aggressive in concert with the application of all that medical technology had to offer. Much touch during this period of time related to medical maintenance of the infant. Jones (1982) noted that premature and ill infants are given general care at rates that may be as much as eight times higher than their full-term healthy peers. Murdoch and Darlow (1984) reported that infants under 1,500 g in their study were the recipients of a mean of 234 procedures per day that involved handling. This translates into the infant being handled approximately once every 6 minutes. Some of this handling is noxious, while other handling involves routine caregiving tasks. However, for the infant with an immature neurologic system, even apparently routine touch can be noxious. One outcome of data related to the frequency of touch is the suggestion that much of the touching and handling in the NICU can be done in clusters spread out at intervals (Lawhorn & Melzar, 1988). Clustering of touch and handling may reduce the adverse effects of handling. The nature of the nursery, the infant's illness, and the need for a variety of medical interventions all mediate against the child's ability to establish behavioral and physiological organization. Thus, the sicker the infant, the more adverse the procedures may become. The result is that the infant is caught in a no-win situation. The child needs medically oriented touch and handling, but it is this very touch/handling that contributes to ongoing disorganization by the infant.

This period (aggressive touch) lasted roughly from the early 1960s into the mid-1980s. The attitude at this time was that the medical community should focus all efforts on saving the baby, with minimal concern directed toward how this aggressive style of intervention affected the surviving infants. The result was that NICUs were largely characterized by too little soothing tactile and kinesthetic touch and by an overabundance of touch associated with pain and discomfort (Catlett & Davis, 1990; Colditz, 1991).

Since the mid-1980s, the concern has shifted more toward the type and quality of touch afforded infants in the NICU. Some descriptive data about touch provided by High and Gorski (1985) offers interesting insights into the amount and type of touch afforded infants in intensive care. The High and Gorski investigation quantified interactions between medical personnel and infants while the infant was in the NICU. Both acutely ill and convalescing infants were observed. A summary of the results revealed the following:

1. *Percentage of time nurse was present:* Nurses were present for only 30% of the time for acutely ill infants and 20% of the time for infants considered to be convalescing.

2. *Percentage of time no caregiver was present:* No caregiver of any kind was present for 63% of the observations of acutely ill infants and for 71% of the observations of convalescent infants. These percentages may reflect staffing patterns that assign several infants (in the convalescent stage) to one nurse following a child's need for critical nursing intervention/care.

3. *Interval between nurse completing a caregiving task and leaving the infant's care area:* Nurses spent 85 seconds for acute and 64 seconds for convalescent groups between completing an intervention and leaving the infant's care area.

4. *Amount and type of handling:* Thirteen percent of total observation time included some form of caregiver touching of infants. For acutely ill infants, most touching involved medical procedures (71%), while a nearly equal amount of

medical and social touching (54% versus 60%) was given to convalescent infants.

These figures underscore the need to direct significant attention to touch and interaction patterns that are more nurturative in nature, both in quantity and type of touch. One attempt to do so was reported by Field et al. (1986). Field and colleagues described the effects of tactile-kinesthetic stimulation on a cohort of preterm infants. The group of infants followed consisted of 40 premature newborns with a mean gestational age of 31 weeks and a mean birth weight of 1,280 g. The intervention provided for these infants consisted of a program of body stroking and passive limb movement for three 15-minute periods per day for a total of 10 days. The infants who received this tactile-kinesthetic intervention exhibited a 47% greater weight gain per day; were more alert and active during behavioral observations; showed more mature habituation, orientation, motor, and range of state behavior; and had hospital stays that were shorter by 6 days. An additional investigation using similar methods demonstrated basically comparable findings (Scafidi et al., 1990). Issues raised in both of these studies included which infants should receive kinesthetic-tactile intervention as described in the investigations, as well as the point at which such intervention should begin.

Hartelius, Rasmussen, Sygehus, and Denmark (1992) describe an investigation designed to monitor the impact of touch on a group of 11 premature infants. Stroking was utilized, with careful monitoring of infant state, respiration, and infant body movements. Results indicate that for the youngest and least mature infants, drastic changes in breathing took place when they were stroked. However, in older, more mature infants, respiration rates changed during stroking (either an increase or decrease), but none of the infants became apneic. For the older infants, patterns of body movements and distress signals were more clearly differentiated. The authors indicate that the overall results of the investigation differed from their initial expectations. They noted that preterm infants found it difficult to tolerate massage, but that positive responses were detected for containment techniques that would not stimulate reflexes. The overall implications of this investigation suggest that touch, if used properly, is a therapeutic tool in the healthy growth and development of preterm infants. In addition, demonstrating touch techniques for parents assists them in understanding the signals infants send that suggest stress and how these signals may be unique to each individual infant.

Any discussion of touch for infants in intensive care usually includes some information about calming techniques. Techniques designed to calm stressed infants have been used in many NICUs to minimize the adverse environmental effects to which the infants are exposed. Although calming techniques have been used for varying amounts of time, systematic study of results is limited. Three basic calming techniques are available in the NICU. These are positioning, swaddling, and nonnutritive sucking. A brief discussion of each follows.

- *Positioning:* Preterm infants generally display reduced muscle tone. As a result, the child is likely to assume extended positions of the limbs from prolonged periods in a supine position. Positioning of the infant should promote the development of flexor tone. It has been suggested that prone positioning may be of benefit to many infants in the NICU (Barb & Lemons, 1989; Fay, 1989). The infant may be positioned lying on one side instead of in a supine position. Rolls may be used to maintain this position. Additional suggestions regarding positioning as a calming technique are provided by Mastropaolo (1992) and Fox and Molesky (1990).
- *Swaddling:* Newborn infants, particularly preterm infants, have consistently demonstrated a low threshold for stimulation. This realization provided the initial impetus for efforts to regulate the environment of the NICU. It has also been known that certain populations of ill infants, particularly prenatally drug-exposed infants, are particularly susceptible to overstimulation. Although swaddling has been used by mothers in various cultures for many years, only recently has the benefit of swaddling for ill infants been explored. Although the literature is not extensive, Mastropaolo (1992) demonstrated that swaddling can result in increased oxygenation and reduced heart rate.
- *Nonnutritive sucking:* A final technique used for calming infants in the NICU is nonnutritive sucking. Caregivers have employed nonnutritive sucking for decades to calm infants in the home setting. Babies routinely use their hands, fingers, pacifiers, or other nondangerous objects in an attempt to calm themselves. Kimble and Dempsey (1992) have suggested that nonnutritive sucking affects sleep, state regulation and arousal, oxygenation, nutrition, and growth. In addition, nonnutritive sucking may have positive benefits in enhancing the process of attachment between mother and infant.

A more recent technique related to touching and tactile-kinesthetic stimulation in the NICU is kangaroo care. In this method, the newborn is wrapped onto the parent's chest. The goal is for as much of the child's skin as possible to be in direct contact with as much of the adult's skin as possible. Typically, the child is held in kangaroo fashion for 30 minutes per day. Kangaroo care has been associated with decreased hospital stay, shorter periods on assisted ventilation, as well as increased states of alertness. Hence, a state of alertness conducive to encouraging socio-communicative development is fostered. Mothers who use this technique appear more inclined to breastfeed. Mothers also indicate an enhanced sense of ownership of the child and his or her care while in the NICU. Ludington, Thompson, and Swinth (1992) discuss the efficacy of kangaroo care with preterm infants. A variety of physiologic measures were made on a group of premature infants who received kangaroo care for a period of 2 to 3 hours immediately following one feeding and preceding the next. Both an experimental and control group of infants were studied. The physiologic measures made included heart rate, periodic breathing, respiratory rate, skin temperature, and apnea/bradycardia episodes. Measures were made approximately 4 days prior to infant discharge from the NICU. The results suggest that healthy transitional (close to discharge) infants readily tolerate 2 to 3 hours of kangaroo care without cardiorespiratory or thermal compromise. In addition, more regular and even breathing patterns and more regular quiet sleep were seen in infants receiving kangaroo care. The authors recommend that kangaroo care be an option in NICU care for medically stable infants. Gale, Franck, and Lund (1993) report results of skin-to-skin holding in intubated infants. One of the main benefits of the skin-to-skin touching in the Gale, Franck, and Lund study was the effect on the parents. Although the infants included in the study demonstrated varying degrees of physiologic stress during transfer from the incubator to the skin-to-skin position, as the infants matured their ability to tolerate this transfer increased. Table 4–11 lists a variety of comments shared by parents following skin-to-skin opportunities afforded them as part of the Gale et al. study.

Social Environment and Intervention in the NICU

Information concerning the social environment of the NICU relates in large measure to observations of caregiver and professional staff interaction with infants. The amount of social contact between infants and adults is reduced because of the precarious state of the NICU infant's health. Nonetheless, alterations can be made in the social context of the NICU that may result in enhanced socio-communicative development. It is imperative that hospital-based early interventionists (particularly

TABLE 4–11   Mothers' and Fathers' Comments about Skin-to-Skin Holding

- "It helped me get through this helpless period."
- "This was the first time I knew the baby was mine."
- "It was the first time I felt sure that I was his mother and the nurses were not."
- "I felt more confident talking to the doctors and asking the nurses questions about my baby."
- "I felt less afraid of my baby, her equipment, and doing care for her."
- "For the first time, I felt like I was doing something for my baby that no one else could do."
- "I felt better about my style of caring for my baby and knew that he would do even better at home."

Adapted from "Skin-to-Skin (Kangaroo) Holding of the Intubated Premature Infant," by G. Gale, L. Franck, and C. Lund, 1993, *Neonatal Network, 12,* p. 49.

those in the NICU) become familiar with issues related to the social conditions of the nursery.

INTERACTIONAL OPPORTUNITIES. The opportunity for adults and infants to interact is sharply reduced in the NICU. Tables 4–12 and 4–13 present a sample of interactional barriers seen in NICUs that can impede effective interaction between parents and the infant. Information presented earlier in this chapter provided the time a caregiver is in social contact with his or her infant. Additional data suggest that there is relatively little social contact between parents and infants during NICU hospitalization. Jones (1982) suggests that up to 90% of the touching a child receives in the NICU comes from individuals other than the child's parents. Additional information suggests that mothers are observed interacting with their NICU-confined infants less than 5% of the time (Linn, Horowitz, Buddin, Leake, & Fox, 1985) during daytime visiting hours. Parents would be less likely to visit during night hours, thus reducing social contact opportunities even more. Jones further indicates that NICU staff are in contact with infants with respiratory distress 22% of the time, those with surgical problems 28.5% of the time, and those with complex medical histories 30.7% of the time. As has been previously noted, premature infants receive little social contact with caregivers, and the contact that is received is primarily medical in nature. Marton, Dawson, and Minde (1980) report that premature infants in one study were the recipients of a little over 8 minutes of contact per hour from NICU staff.

TABLE 4–12   Interactional Difficulties in the NICU

Parent Interactional Difficulties
  Stress
  Emotional reactions
  Altered roles in caregiving
  Psychological well-being
  Degree of available social support

Infant Interactional Difficulties
  Medical status
  Degree of prematurity
  Feeding issues
  Neurological integrity

NICU Environment: Barriers to Interaction
  Noncontingent stimulation
  Ongoing medical interventions
  Noxious environmental stimuli
  Lack of privacy
  General flow of activity in the NICU

Adapted from "Parent-Infant Interaction in Neonatal Intensive Care Units: Implications for Research and Service Delivery," by S. Gottwald and S. Thurman, 1990, *Infants and Young Children, 2*, p. 1.

TABLE 4–13   Barriers to Parenting in the NICU

Physical	*Psychological/Emotional*
Unit space	Lack of privacy
Parent accommodation	Feelings of inadequacy, guilt, and
Distance from home	helplessness
	Loss of control
	Fear of attachment
Mechanical	*Unit/Health Care*
Professionals	Policies and standards
Respiratory equipment	Staffing patterns
Phototherapy	Nonsupportive work setting
Infant beds	Emotions/values/culture
Invasive equipment	Personal relationship with the infant

Adapted from "The Evolution of Parental Roles in the NICU," by K. Plaas, 1994, *Neonatal Network, 13*, p. 31.

Differences have also been observed between mothers and fathers regarding social interaction with their children during NICU experiences. Several investigators have reported that mothers talk to their infants more than fathers during NICU visits. Additionally, data suggests that infants in intensive care behave differently toward their mothers and fathers. Fathers have been reported as being more disengaged from their infants during visits. It has been indicated that fathers interact with their infants in a more remote fashion than mothers. Mothers are generally more affectionate. It has also been noted that both mothers and fathers communicate more with their child during NICU visits when they are visiting individually, rather than as a couple (Marton, Minde, & Perotta, 1981; Thurman & Korteland, 1989). Overall parental visits may be infrequent, depending on the individual family situation, distance from the NICU, and finances. Parental visits to the NICU during the initial part of a child's hospitalization may be characterized as less active and interactive and also generally tenuous in nature. During early visits, parents may be more inclined to simply look at their child than to attempt to interact with the child. It is imperative that the EI alert the parents to the states premature infants display during their NICU stay. Parents can be encouraged to persevere in their attempts to interact with their child. They should be told that once the child gains a measure of better health, enhanced interaction opportunities will take place. Parents can also be alerted to the variety of behavioral responses their child will display while in the hospital. Table 4–14 presents examples of behavioral responses infants in intensive care are likely to display. It is imperative that the EI alert parents and caregivers to this range of behaviors, as well as to the significance of the behaviors observed. Later sensitivity to infant-initiated communicative signals may, at least in part, be related to the degree to which the parents are able to identify early communicative signals such as those listed in Table 4–14. This is a significant area of need and one in which the EI can be of immeasurable help to the parents. Adults will devote significant effort toward establishing interactions with their child, providing the adult receives some degree of payback for these efforts. Parents of children in intensive care often display patterns of discouragement when they are unable to engage in interactions with their sick child. They often report that one of the hardest things to adjust to is the feeling that their child does not know that they are there (present in the nursery). It is imperative that they be informed that the child does know they are there, but because of the child's current health status, he is not able to provide them with any consistent awareness of the parents' presence.

TABLE 4–14   Examples of Behavioral
Responses

Stress and Defense Behaviors

Autonomic and Visceral Signs
   Hiccuping
   Yawning

Motoric Stress Signs
   Motoric flaccidity
   Motoric hypertonicity
   Frantic, diffuse activity

State-Related Stress Signals
   Eye floating
   Strained fussiness or crying

Self-Regulatory and Approach Behaviors

Autonomic Stability
   Smooth respiration
   Pink, stable color

Motoric Stability
   Smooth, well-modulated posture
   Well-regulated tone

State Stability and Attentional Regulation
   Clear, robust sleep states
   Reliable consolability

Adapted from "A Synactive Model of Neonatal Behavior Organization: Framework for the Assessment
of Neurobehavioral Development in the Preterm Infant and for the Support of Infants and Parents in
the Neonatal Intensive Care Environment," by H.
Als, 1986, *Physical and Occupational Therapy in
Pediatrics, 6*, p. 3.

Socio-communication-based interaction. Jacobsen and Wendler (1988)
provide insightful information on the amount of language interactions nurses in the NICU displayed with infants. The investigation
was designed to measure the number of opportunities nurses had to
speak to infants and the actual talking that took place. Using an alter-
nating time sampling method of observation, a total of 1,200 time
intervals were observed in the NICU. Of the 1,200 observations, the
investigators determined that language-based interaction was possi-

ble 385 times. Of these 385 opportunities when language-based interaction was possible, nurses actually talked to the infants 47 times. The
implication is quite clear. Nursing staff do not take advantage of a
significant number of language interaction opportunities. The authors
noted that the opportunity to talk to infants appeared to be related, at
least in part, to nursing routine. Nursing responsibilities such as
charting and checking equipment certainly place heavy obligations on
the nurses' time. However, the small amount of talking that did take
place, when compared to the number of opportunities when talking
could have taken place, provides ready suggestions about the social
environment of the NICU.

In an additional investigation, Jacobsen, Starnes, and Gasser (1998)
examined the effectiveness of an in-hospital training program
designed to increase mothers' production of descriptions and praises
directed toward their infants. This study was predicated on the realization that preterm infants are at enhanced risk for communication
delay and subsequent risk for school failure. The mothers in the experimental group were provided with a list of 50 utterances linked to
descriptions of the infants' behavior, as well as an additional 50 utterances related to praises of infants' behavior. Table 4–15 lists a sample
of the descriptions and praises the mothers were exposed to.
Following the mothers' exposure to these utterances (both descriptions
and praises), measures of maternal generalization were made.
Following the training, mothers significantly increased their frequency of generalizations and praises of their babies' behaviors. Mothers
were again measured 1 month following the child's discharge from the
NICU. It was particularly encouraging to note that mothers maintained these interaction skills. The implications for long-term enhancement of communication skills are apparent. It is reasonable to assume
that long-term follow-up of communication skills for the infants and
mothers who participated in this investigation may likely reveal
greater communication skills than would be observed in infants and
mothers in the control group. This investigation demonstrates that
even relatively short-term communication-based NICU intervention,
directed toward caregivers, has the potential for long-term enhancement of communication skills.

Home-Based Early Intervention Services

Evaluations of early intervention programs that incorporate home visiting demonstrate that home visiting programs can improve both the

TABLE   4–15 Sample of
Mothers' Descriptions and Praises and Reinforcers

Maternal Descriptions

- You opened your eyes.
- You're sucking your thumb.
- You're sleepy.
- You look happy today.
- You look tired.
- You have two ears.
- You look cold.
- Your legs are so tiny.
- You're wet.
- You have 10 toes.

Maternal Praises

- You're such a good baby.
- You are growing so fast.
- Mommy loves you.
- I like the way you smile.
- You are my favorite baby.
- You're doing so well.
- I like the way you stretch.
- You have such cute toes.
- You'll be a big boy/girl.

Verbal Reinforcements for Mothers

- I like the way you said that.
- You're doing it.
- That is good
  describing/praising.
- That is what I want you to do.
- That's great; keep it up.
- Good job Mrs..
- You're such a talker.

Adapted from "An Experimental Analysis
of the Generalization of Descriptions and
Praises for Mothers of Premature Infants," by C. Jacobsen, C. Starnes, and
V. Gasser, 1988, *Human Communication Canada, 12,* p. 23.

short- and long-term health and well-being of families and children. In addition, evaluations of the cost of home visiting early intervention programs have demonstrated that long-term savings are realized for those children in need of special services designed to optimize later school performance. In other words, home-based early intervention improves child and family outcome and saves money.

Home-based services are defined as those in which infants, toddlers, and their families with special needs receive early intervention assistance in the home through home visiting professionals representing one or more early intervention disciplines. Of necessity, a transdisciplinary approach toward services delivered in the home must be employed. It is not possible, from a time and cost standpoint, for a multitude of early intervention experts to visit a home. Hence, home visiting early intervention specialists must bring a variety of skills and experiences into their role as home visitor, while at the same time realizing their limitations in crossing disciplinary boundaries.

Home visiting is not a new concept. Home-based services for medically fragile adults have been available for some time. However, the concept of home-based early intervention for infants is a more recent application of a home-based model of service delivery. The primary advantage to the child and family of home visiting is that needed services are provided in the most natural of all settings, the home. A substantial growth in home-based early intervention programs has been noted in the past 15 years. Wasik and Roberts (1989) suggest that literally thousands of home visiting programs exist in the United States. Roberts and Wasik (1990) report that in a 1990 survey of early intervention programs (1,904 home visit programs), 34% reported serving children from birth to age 3 years. The children served received services for developmental delay, physical handicap, specific learning impairment, low birth weight, or other risk factors. Home visiting is a flexible and cost-effective strategy for providing services to infants, toddlers, and their families. In existing home visiting programs, there are a variety of formats related to curriculum, emphasis, the occupation of the EI making the home visit, the intensity of visits, and populations served. No single model of home visiting has been consistently demonstrated to be the most effective. Issues of distance (geography), availability of EI personnel, funding, and other service needs surface as home-based intervention services are instituted in a community. The general philosophy behind home visiting is that at-risk infants and families, especially those who are poor, uneducated, or headed by teenage parents, often face significant barriers in accessing the early intervention services they need. Home visiting can reduce these barriers.

Filler (1983) lists several benefits for a home-based model of early intervention. These are modified as follows:

1. Parents feel more comfortable in their own home and, therefore, act more naturally.

2. Similarly, children are more likely to perform better in their own home. It affords a more naturalistic setting in which to elicit behaviors and provide intervention activities.

3. A child's health is better protected. This may be of particular importance for those children who are medically fragile.

4. Parent and child routines are not interrupted. As a result, a more accurate sample of parent-child routines may be observed.

5. There is a greater likelihood of gaining helpful insights because other family members are present.

The experienced early interventionist soon comes to realize that the benefits of home visiting as an early intervention strategy coexist with certain liabilities. Although the discussion that follows is not exhaustive, it should serve to alert the home visiting EI to several possible pitfalls.

First, the home visiting EI must be alert to the potential for a wide range of responses and interactions by the family during the visit. These responses may include an extreme degree of comfort on the part of the caregivers, resulting in the EI being ignored and leading to a response pattern in which the parents hand the child to the "professional" and relinquish their responsibilities as primary caregivers during the visit. On the opposite end of the continuum is a response pattern in which hostility is expressed toward the EI. This hostility can emanate from a variety of sources. However, a primary source of hostility in instances such as this relates to the caregivers' lack of acceptance of the unique needs their child has. These response patterns are inappropriate and counterproductive to effective home-based early intervention services. Finally, many EIs provide home-based intervention services in large metropolitan areas across the United States and genuine concern for personal safety becomes a significant issue. The early interventionist providing services in the home environment must always keep in mind that those services are dispensed on someone else's "turf" and that there are cautions inherent in operating in a home setting. An additional consideration relates to the need for effective communication between professionals, particularly if more than one is providing services in the home. It is possible, for example, for two or more EI professionals to visit the home. It is also possible that EIs visiting the home work for different agencies. Thus, communication between home visitors is difficult. In instances of this nature, it is advised that a EI log be left at the home. Through use of the EI log, each EI can provide the others with information relating to the services each individual is providing. More recently, an increasing number of states are moving toward a total home-based model of service delivery for children under 3 years of age. In these instances, all services are delivered in the home setting only. The final chapter in this text presents detailed information related to the efficacy of home visiting as an early intervention service delivery model.

Combination Home-Center Settings

Effective early intervention services can be delivered through combination home-based and center-based programs. Although there is no set format for such intervention, a child's individual needs may serve to dictate the exact nature of the home-center combination of services provided. The Infant Health and Development Program (1990) demonstrated an intervention approach that provided home-based services up to a child's first birthday and center-based services after that. Combination home-center programs may fit best for children with specific educational and/or health needs. This model offers the advantages of both center- and home-based intervention. Center-based settings often provide a home-based intervention program initially. Once the child is settled in the home and the caregivers have made proper hospital-to-home adjustments, a center-based component may be added.

Regardless of which model is used, several conditions are needed in any early intervention setting. First, during the time of medical or specialized care, opportunities for normal experience should be afforded each child when possible. Second, parents must be considered as full partners in all decision making. And third, a primary goal of the intervention program should be the movement of the child to a less restricted environment, whatever that might be.

ONSET AND FREQUENCY OF INTERVENTION SERVICES

A logical question in any early intervention program relates to when services should begin and how frequently intervention services should be provided. One important concept to keep in mind is that, regardless of the setting in which services are provided, the caregivers are full partners and part of the comprehensive intervention program designed for their child. As such, intervention in one sense takes place all the time. As parents learn how to take advantage of naturally occurring events in the life of the family for the purpose of attaining intervention goals, a case can be made that intervention never ends.

Prevention is always preferable to rehabilitation. Hence, the earlier a child is identified and the earlier intervention is begun, the greater the developmental gains that are noted and the less the likelihood of later problems. Earlier is better. One problem in fully implementing the philosophy "earlier is better" lies in the reality that many early intervention programs require that a child's delay be manifested prior to the initiation of intervention services. This is a mistake because valuable intervention time is lost while the intervention team waits for the child's delay to progress to the point that it is more readily quantified through infant-toddler assessment. This is not to suggest that each child with a hint of risk should be included in early intervention. Rather, it is to suggest that a balance point must be reached relative to the child's manifestation of measurable delay and the child's display of risk factors that in all likelihood will lead to measurable delay if intervention services are not begun.

Although the concept of "earlier is better" applies to age of identification and initiation of intervention services, a corollary concept of "more is better" may not be as applicable. The intensity (frequency) of intervention must be carefully matched to meet each child's and family's needs. Intervention planners should never lose sight of the overall adjustments the family and child must make. It is easy for caregivers to assume, based on their intense desire to do all that is possible for their child, that they must be in constant motion, running the child from therapist to therapist and from intervention activity to intervention activity. Bryant and Graham (1993) have noted that the intensity of early intervention services must be defined according to the purpose of the service, the level of expertise required, and the overall amount of services required. They further suggest that the question of how much service is needed for a particular child can be answered only by addressing all variables, including the child's developmental needs, health-related concerns, additional supports needed by the family, and the overall availability of required intervention services. This can be a difficult balancing act for the EI and caregivers. However, it must be constantly kept in mind that decisions about intensity of services must be made as a result of a full partnership between EI professionals and caregivers.

A review of literature on actual intervention "contact time" suggests that those programs that provide increased contact time (within the limits and overall considerations previously indicated) generally tend to be more successful than programs with less contact time. Recent evaluation of home visiting programs that studied amount of contact time demonstrated that weekly versus biweekly home visits produced greater child change (Powell & McGregor, 1989).

CHAPTER SUMMARY

This chapter was intended to alert the EI to a host of issues related to communication-based early intervention services. These services may be initiated in the intensive care nursery and continue after the child transitions to the home setting. It is imperative that the EI recall the principle of continuum of risk. This concept implies that the seeds for school failure begin, for many children, quite early. Hence, early identification and initiation of intervention services serve to reduce and/or ameliorate later delay. Thus for many children, school failure is prevented rather than rehabilitated at a later date. The cost benefits alone of this approach make early identification and intervention of significant benefit. All members of the early intervention team, including the caregivers, must become familiar with the issues raised in this chapter. The ultimate beneficiaries of these suggestions will be the children served.

REFERENCES

Als, H. (1986). A synactive model of neonatal behavioral organization: Framework for the assessment of neurobehavioral development in the preterm infant and for the support of infants and parents in the neonatal intensive care environment. *Physical and Occupational Therapy in Pediatrics, 6*, 3.

Barb, S., & Lemons, P. (1989). The premature infant: Toward improving neurodevelopmental outcome. *Neonatal Network, 7*, 7.

Barker, A. (1991, March). The transition home for preterm infants: Parents' perceptions. *Neonatal Network, 4*, 50.

Bryant, D., & Graham, M. (Eds.).(1983). *Implementing early intervention.* New York: Guilford Press.

Capute, A., Palmer, F., & Shapiro, B. (1987). Using language to track development. *Patient Care, 11*, 60.

Catlett, A., & Davis, P. (1990). Environmental stimulation of the acutely ill premature infant: Physiological effects and nursing implications. *Neonatal Network, 8*, 19.

Colditz, P. (1991). Review article: Management of pain in the newborn infant. *Journal of Pediatric Child Health, 27*, 11.

Dunn, S., van Kleek, A., & Rossetti, L. (1993). Current roles and continuing needs of speech-language pathologists working in neonatal intensive care units. *American Journal of Speech-Language Pathology, 1*, 25.

Fay, M. (1989). The positive effects of positioning. *Neonatal Network, 6*, 23.

Fenichel, E., & Eggbeer, L. (1991). Preparing practitioners to work with infants, toddlers, and their families: Four essential elements of training. *Infants and Young Children, 4*, 56.

Field, T., Schanberg, S., Scafidi, F., Bauer, C., Vega, N., Garcia, R., Nystrum, J., & Kuhn, C. (1986). Tactile/kinesthetic stimulation effect on preterm neonates. *Pediatrics, 77*, 654.

Filler, J. (1983). Service models for handicapped infants. In S. Gray Garwood & R. Fewell (Eds.), *Educating handicapped infants* (p. 185). Rockville, MD: Aspen.

Fox, M., & Molesky, M. (1990). The effects of prone and supine positioning on arterial oxygen pressure. *Neonatal Network, 8*, 25.

Gale, G., Franck, L., & Lund, C. (1993). Skin-to-skin (kangaroo) holding of the intubated premature infant. *Neonatal Network, 12*, 49.

Gennaro, S., Brooten, D., & Bakewell-Sachs, S. (1991). Post-discharge services for low birth-weight infants. *Journal of Neonatal Nursing, 11*, 29.

Glass, P., Avery, G., Subramanian, K., Keys, M., Sostek, A., & Friendly, D. (1985). Effect of bright light in the hospital on incidence of retinopathy of prematurity. *New England Journal of Medicine, 313*, 401.

Gleich, M. (1942). The premature infant: Part 3. *Archives of Pediatrics, 59*, 172.

Gottfried, A. (1985). Environment of newborn infants in special care units. In A. Gottfried & J. Gaiter (Eds.), *Infant stress under intensive care: Environmental neonatology* (p. 55). Baltimore: University Park Press.

Gottwald, S., & Thurman, S. (1990). Parent-infant interaction in neonatal intensive care units: Implications for research and service delivery. *Infants and Young Children, 2*, 1.

Hanson, M., & Brekken, L. (1991). Early intervention personnel model and standards: An interdisciplinary field-developed approach. *Infants and Young Children, 4*, 54.

Hartelius, I., Rasmussen, L., Sygehus, O., & Denmark, O. (1992). How little you are! *Neonatal Network, 11*, 33.

Hayes, M., & Ensher, G. (1994). Intervening in intensive care nurseries. In G. Ensher & D. Clark (Eds.), *Newborns at risk* (p. 227). Gaithersburg, MD: Aspen Press.

High, P., & Gorski, P. (1985). Recording environmental influences on infant development in the intensive care nursery: Womb for improvement. In A. Gottfried & J. Gaiter (Eds.), *Infant stress under intensive care* (p. 200). Baltimore: University Park Press.

Infant Health and Development Program (IHDP). (1990). Enhancing the outcomes of low birth-weight, premature infants. *Journal of the American Medical Association, 263*, 3035.

Jacobsen, C., Starnes, C., & Gasser, V. (1988). An experimental analysis of the generalization of descriptions and praises for mothers of premature infants. *Human Communication Canada, 12,* 23–33.

Jacobsen, C., & Wendler, S. (1988). Language stimulation in the neonatal intensive care unit. *Human Communication Canada, 12,* 48.

Jones, C. (1982). Environmental analysis of neonatal intensive care. *Journal of Nervous and Mental Disease, 170,* 144.

Katz, K., Pokorni, J., & Long, T. (1989). *Chronically ill and at-risk infants: Family centered intervention from hospital to home.* Palo Alto, CA: Vort Corporation.

Kimble, C., & Dempsey, J. (1992). Nonnutritive sucking: Adaptation and health for the neonate. *Neonatal Network, 11,* 29.

Largo, R., Molinari, L., Pinto, L., & Weber, C. (1986). Language development of term and preterm children during the first five years of life. *Developmental Medicine and Child Neurology, 28,* 333.

Lawhorn, G., & Melzar, A. (1988). Developmental care for the very low birth weight infant. *Journal of Perinatal Neonatal Nursing, 2,* 56.

Linn, P., Horowitz, F., Buddin, B., Leake, J., & Fox, H. (1985). An ecological description of a neonatal intensive care unit. In A. Gottfried & J. Gaiter (Eds.), *Infant stress under intensive care: Environmental neonatology* (p. 190). Baltimore: University Park Press.

Lockwood, S. (1994). Early speech and language indicators for later learning problems: Recognizing a language organization disorder. *Infants and Young Children, 7,* 43.

Long, J., Lucey, J., & Philip, A. (1980). Excessive handling as a cause of hypoxemia. *Pediatrics, 65,* 203.

Ludington, S., Thompson, C., & Swinth, J. (1992). Efficacy of kangaroo care with preterm infants in open-air cribs. *Neonatal Network, 11,* 101.

Marton, P. Dawson, H., & Minde, K. (1980). The interaction of ward personnel with infants in the premature nursery. *Infant Behavior and Development, 3,* 307.

Marton, P., Minde, K., & Perotta, M. (1981). The role of the father of the infant at risk. *Infant Behavior and Development, 51,* 672.

Mastropaolo, A. (1992). *The at risk infant: Medical insult and intervention.* Unpublished lecture, Syracuse University, Syracuse, NY.

McWilliam, R., & Strain, P. (1993). Service delivery models in DEC recommended practices: Indicators of quality in programs for infants and young children with special needs and their families. Reston, VA: Council for Exceptional Children.

Murdoch, D., & Darlow, B. (1984). Handling during neonatal intensive care. *Archives of Disease in Childhood, 59,* 957.

Peabody, J., & Lewis, K. (1985). Consequences of neonatal intensive care. In A. Gottfried & J. Gaiter (Eds.), *Infant stress under intensive care* (p. 180). Baltimore: University Park Press.

Plaas, K. (1994). The evolution of parental roles in the NICU. *Neonatal Network, 13,* 31.

Powell, C., & McGregor, S. (1989). Home visiting of varying frequency and child development. *Pediatrics, 84,* 157.

Roberts, R., & Wasik, B. (1990). Home visiting programs for families with children birth to three: Results of a national survey. *Journal of Early Intervention, 14,* 274.

Rowan, L., Thorpe, E., & McCollum, J. (1990). An interdisciplinary practicum to foster infant-family and teaming competencies in speech-language pathologists. *Infants and Young Children, 2,* 58.

Scafidi, F., Field, T., Schanberg, S., Bauer, C., Tucci, K., Roberts, J., Morrow, C., & Kuhn, C. (1990). *Infant Behavior and Development, 13,* 167.

Schultz, M. (1987). Hearing screening. In H. Taeusch & M. Yogman (Eds.), *Follow-up management of the high-risk infant* (p. 310). Boston: Little, Brown.

Thurman, S., & Korteland, C. (1989). The behavior of mothers and fathers toward their infants during neonatal intensive care visits. *Children's Health Care, 18,* 247.

VandenBerg, K. (1993). Basic competencies to begin developmental care in the intensive care nursery. *Infants and Young Children, 6,* 52.

Wasik, B., & Roberts, R. (1989). Home visiting with low income families. *Family Resource Coalition Report, 9,* 8.

Wolke, D. (1987). Environmental and developmental neonatology. *Journal of Reproductive and Infant Psychology, 5,* 17.

APPENDIX 4-A: CURRICULA/MATERIALS FOR COMMUNICATION-BASED INTERVENTION

Devine, M. (1990). *Growing together: Communication activities for infants and toddlers*. Tucson, AZ: Communication Skill Builders. (Books 1 to 3 cover activities from birth through 36 months of age.)

Furno, S. (1993). *Helping babies learn*. Tucson, AZ: Communication Skill Builders.

Johnson, K., & Heinze, B. (1990). *Hickory dickory talk: A family approach to infant and toddler language development*. East Moline, IL: LinguiSystems.

Linder, T. (1993). *Transdisciplinary play-based intervention*. Baltimore: Paul H. Brookes.

Manolson, A. (1992). *It takes two to talk*. Toronto, Canada: Hanen Center Publication.

Niemeyer, S. (1994). *Caregiver education guide for children with developmental disabilities*. Gaithersburg, MD: Aspen Press.

Weitzman, E. (1992). *Learning language and loving it*. Toronto, Canada: Hanen Center Publication.

CASE STUDY

In an attempt to acquaint clinicians with a likely scenario for a child in the NICU as well as the services (developmental care) the child may receive, the following case study is presented. Although this case study may not be typical of all NICUs or early intervention opportunities, it does have similarities to what would be available to a child in most locations in the United States.

Thomas was born at 27 weeks' gestation weighing 780 g, thus placing him in the small-for-gestational-age category. He is the only child of Betsy, a 23-year-old mother, and Philip, her husband. Thomas sustained a grade II intercranial hemorrhage, required 17 days of assisted ventilation, suffered intermittent seizures, and remained in an in-turned state until he was 26 days of age. Both Betsy and Philip spent as much time in the NICU as possible. Betsy was given regular opportunity to assist with Thomas' care. She participated in tasks such as bathing and changing his position and was permitted to write her observations in a special section of the child's hospital chart. She was also asked to complete a developmental care plan, with assistance from nurses, at least every other day. During Thomas' stay in the NICU, he transitioned to the coming-out state and showed initial awareness of his surroundings and people at approximately 24 to 26 days of age. When he began to come out, this was carefully explained to Betsy, and she was encouraged to be there as much as possible. She was most willing to do so.

Thomas' overall developmental care plan called for frequent changes in position, reduction of noise, no direct overhead lighting, minimal handling (during the first 21 days), and clustering of medical care (clustering medical procedures closely so that the child is not stressed throughout the day). Betsy experienced several significant bouts of anxiety, particularly during the early days of his hospital stay. There were times when her frustration centered around the statement, "He does not know that I am here." It was explained to Betsy that Thomas did know she was there, but he was not yet able to give her any of the typical "Gerber baby" responses. She was permitted to stroke his legs and rub his head. When she did this, Thomas' respiratory rate and oxygen level changed slightly. This was enough for Betsy because she said, "Yes, he does know I am here."

The hospital's decision to enlist her assistance in providing very basic care for Thomas eased her anxiety because she was allowed to feel that she had a role in his care. There were several instances in which she felt that the staff was not listening to her or not answering her questions fully. She directed anger toward several staff members on one or two occasions. On each occasion she apologized to the staff involved and explained that her behavior was due to fear for Thomas' survival.

Philip was encouraged to be involved in Thomas' care as much as possible. He was asked to assist in changing position and some routine caregiving tasks. He was somewhat reluctant and fearful to do so but did respond with some prompting and encouragement. Neither Betsy nor Philip had extended family in the community; thus they had minimal support from others. Although they had regular communication with their parents, neither set of grandparents was able to assist Philip and Betsy.

Once Thomas transitioned into the coming-out state, more intentional interactional opportunities were explored. He began to eat primarily by mouth (with the assistance of the feeding specialist in the NICU). The feeding specialist took great care in educating Betsy, and as soon as possible Betsy assumed increased responsibility for feeding Thomas. She was quite hesitant initially but quickly learned that she could be successful in feeding him.

At this point (within 3 days of feeding by mouth), Thomas began to display increased periods of alertness. He began to show awareness of others and more consistently responded when he was spoken to. As he gained weight, his periods of alertness increased in frequency and length. Betsy was introduced to kangaroo care, to which she took immediately. Her response upon first feeling Thomas' skin on hers was one of joy, appreciation, and some anxiety. Philip also participated in kangaroo care; however, he was more reluctant and tentative. Philip did not feed Thomas during hospitalization. From day 34 on, Thomas steadily gained weight and was free from additional medical complications. He was dismissed to the home setting on day 47.

A social worker and the feeding specialist home-monitored Thomas' transition. The developmental specialist took care in explaining that Thomas was at increased risk for health and developmental concerns. It was explained to the parents that Thomas should be monitored carefully to identify and detect any delay in development. They understood that it was imperative that Thomas be enrolled in the developmental follow-up clinic.

When Thomas was 6 months old, it was determined that he was displaying a general delay in motor development, and referral to the community early intervention program was initiated. Thomas received home-based early intervention services once a week for 8 months. While the primary focus of intervention was directed toward motor skills, the physical therapist providing the services also demonstrated how Betsy might enhance Thomas' communication skills. Betsy was shown, initially by the physical therapist and later by the speech-language pathologist, how to initiate turn-taking exchanges with Thomas. In addition, Betsy was shown how to read Thomas' communication signals. These included the manner in which he widened his eyes, coordinated respiration to voice, and "requested" interaction with Betsy. Thomas slowly demonstrated an increase in age-appropriate developmental skill mastery. He is now 23 months of age. His communication skills continue to lag slightly behind age expectations, but he is a communicator and continues to make progress. It is anticipated that Thomas will demonstrate school readiness by school age. It is unknown whether additional services will be needed once he reaches 3 years of age.

Observations

1. Thomas' parents were provided sufficient support, information, and responsibility during his stay in the NICU.

2. Betsy, in particular, was encouraged to participate in a portion of his direct care while he was hospitalized. This made her feel that she was an important part of his care, that her input was needed; and that she could, upon discharge, meet his needs.

3. Betsy and Philip were informed that hospital discharge does not mean that their vigilance for Thomas was over. They were informed that he was at increased risk for developmental delay and that he needed to be monitored carefully to identify any areas of delay as early as possible.

4. During hospitalization Betsy was put in contact with other mothers who had similar experiences in the NICU.

5. Once an area of delay was identified, Thomas was immediately referred for early intervention. The model employed (home-based; transdisciplinary) was reflective of best practice and tailored to meet his individual needs.

6. Regular reassessment was provided. This enabled the EI professionals to monitor his developmental change and make adjustments as needed.

7. The entire early intervention team (school readiness) agreed upon long-term objectives. The team identified motor skills as the initial area on which to focus. Later, communication skills were stressed.

8. The parents were made aware of the potential need of continuing services for Thomas between the ages of 3 to 5 years.

CHAPTER
5

Keep the Conversation Going: Specific Strategies for Communication-Based Intervention

❝ *Children do not acquire effective communication skills in a laboratory. Rather, they master the ability to communicate through naturalistic interactions with their world. This mechanism involves learning how to engage in conversations with others. Hence, dialogue skills (becoming a conversationalist) are the centerpiece for communication development. It is therefore necessary that caregivers and clinicians embrace the philosophy that the most effectual intervention strategy for children with communication delay is to* **keep the conversation going. ❞**

The intervention suggestions in this chapter are predicated on two very simple yet important concepts. First, no matter how skilled the early interventionist may be and no matter how much experience the EI may have in providing communication-based intervention, the EI is functioning as a substitute for nature. In other words, if nature did its job, the EI would not have one. This is a somewhat humbling concept but true nonetheless. The second concept flows from the first. That is, no matter how skilled or experienced the

EI may be, one can never beat nature. In other words, to bypass the naturalistic manner in which children acquire communication skills is to set the stage for failure. It can be argued with some force that, from a historical perspective, previous attempts to structure intervention activities for children displaying delayed communication skills tended to place substantial emphasis on the scientific basis of language learning and behavior rather than on the naturalistic manner in which children acquire communication skills (see Table 5–1). Historically, communication interventionists have focused primarily on syntactic, morphological, and semantic aspects of communication/language learning as targets for early intervention. Communication-based intervention focused mainly on teaching grammatical relationships between component parts of language form. The assumption was that once these forms were taught, the learner would generalize to other communication contexts. This did not take place to the degree anticipated, and interventionists have been forced to rethink their approach toward communication-based intervention. As a result, the hub of intervention has shifted away from communicative form and more toward communicative function.

For example, Table 5–1 lists characteristics of typical mother-infant communication. Two of these are worth mentioning at this point. Clinical implications and suggestions for each will be presented later in this chapter.

- *Short utterance length with simple syntax:* Before they are about 5 to 7 months of age, infants are primarily interested in faces. After that age they become primarily interested in objects. Primary interest in objects takes place at about the time the child gains voluntary reach and grasp. Further, infants re-

TABLE 5–1   Characteristics of Typical Mother-Infant Communication

- Short utterance length with simple syntax
- Small core vocabulary—object centered
- Topics limited to the here and now
- Heightened facial expression and gesture
- Frequent questioning and greeting
- Meaningful responses—turn taking and prolonging
- Frequent verbal rituals

spond best to utterances that are produced at an even cadence with a wide inflectional pattern. Optimal utterance
length designed to gain infant attention should be 4 to 7
words. Infants have been shown, from an early age, to coor-
dinate arm, leg, eye, and respiratory effort to the cadence of
the adult's speech. In addition, up to 5 to 7 months of age the
child is the primary initiator of communication interactions,
but the adult can prolong the interaction. After that point the
adult and infant will initiate and prolong equally. These observations give rise to several very practical intervention suggestions that will be developed fully later in this chapter.

- *Frequent verbal rituals:* Caregivers of typically developing
children under the age of 3 years generally agree that there
are several daily caregiving tasks that tend to be stressful.
Parents report that dressing, bathing, eating, and bedtime
can be difficult times during the day. In response, many caregivers develop (unplanned and unrehearsed) ritualistic
games that prove to be fun for the child and help ease them
through the caregiving task at hand. Games that surround
bathing and eating are common. These verbal rituals are rich
in communication, language, and conversational activities. It
has been my observation, however, that up to 75% of caregivers of children with special needs never develop verbal
rituals as part of their daily routine. Their attention is focused
on completing a specific task, and they have not developed
mutually pleasurable verbal rituals. This is a simple observation but one that has significant implications. In those instances where verbal rituals are absent, the EI may demonstrate several to parents. See Table 5–1 for a more complete
listing of the characteristics of mother-infant communication.

Neither of the above examples are based on the traditional view
presented by language science, but rather spring from a more naturalistic view of communication development.

The preceding discussion was not meant to suggest that a scientific base for understanding language acquisition and performance is
not important. It is to suggest, however, that children have been
acquiring communication skills quite nicely without the benefit of a
vast scientific understanding of how the process takes place. In other
words, the EI is encouraged to return to what nature has shown to be
valid rather than employ a particular model of intervention because it
fits one's choice of language learning theories. The science of lan-

guage learning and performance has a powerful place in structuring intervention activities. However, a particular model should not be elevated above what the natural course of nature dictates. We can't beat nature, so let's not try, particularly for the populations of children described in previous chapters.

Wilcox (1989) has suggested that children displaying early communication delays or disorders do not simply outgrow these difficulties. In addition, Wilcox indicates that communication problems persist and are related to subsequent academic and social difficulties or deficits. The relationship between early and later disabilities is known to present a significant barrier to educational placement and progress. As stated elsewhere, communication skills are highly predictive of school success. Hence, it is imperative that all EI professionals understand the importance of early communication-based intervention and that this intervention mirror a naturalistic model of communication development.

One key component inherent in the following intervention suggestions is the involvement of the caregivers as communication intervention participants. An entire section of this chapter is devoted to assisting parents as communication facilitators.

It should be recalled that children come into the world uniquely predisposed to learn to communicate. More specifically, children come into the world uniquely predisposed to consume and make sense of it. In most instances, nothing special has to be done. Assuming that the child is healthy and presents no specific sensory deficits, all the child needs is sufficient exposure to his or her language environment and nature does the rest. A child's unique drive to get to know the world is evidenced in a number of ways.

Two important observations gleaned from the human development literature underscore this. First, children are uniquely alert and attuned to the world for the first few hours after birth, assuming a healthy delivery. In other words, there is such a thing as a "sensitive period." This is a period of time in which newborns are specially attuned to their new environment. Second, mothers the world over are exceptionally interested in making contact with their newborns. Regardless of language, culture, or birthing practices, mothers basically say the same thing after the birth of their child. They ask, immediately following the child's birth, "Can I see him?" or "Let me look at her." Hence, the process of socio-communicative development begins early, with significant potential for disruption for the ill infant. Early mother-infant communication provides the foundation for evolving communication skills. In other words, prelinguistic communication development begins very early—shortly after birth. Hence, attention must be directed toward activities that can augment prelinguistic development.

PRELINGUISTIC COMMUNICATION INTERVENTION

Before the emergence of a child's first purposeful word, a number of prelinguistic components to communication must take place. Interaction, attachment, play, pragmatics, and gesture are all important aspects in the development of age-appropriate communication skills. Prelinguistic communication is the child's intentional communication behaviors that do not involve words. Although adults may attribute communicative value to some early behaviors exhibited by a child, actions such as crying when hungry or in pain are not intentional communicative attempts. In the context of the discussion that follows, intentional communication is any behavior directed to an adult or caregiver that conveys information or has some pragmatic function (Weatherby, Cain, Yonclas, & Walker, 1988). The relationship between delayed prelinguistic communication development and linguistic communication development is well established. A greater understanding of prelinguistic intervention activities can increase the benefit of subsequent linguistic intervention. As Yoder and Warren (1993) have suggested, there are essentially two main reasons why targeting prelinguistic development early in the intervention process results in elevated linguistic development. First, enhancing the child's use of vocalization and intentional communication should serve to lay a foundation for better use of adult input in the language development process. And second, as the child's frequency and clarity of communication improve, additional adult-child interactions (turn taking) emerge. The result is improved overall language performance. As Yoder and Warren (1993) suggest, several potential prelinguistic intervention approaches are available to the EI. This discussion is not meant to be exhaustive, but rather to reflect a sampling of current thinking about intervention methods.

One tactic has the adult looking for and participating in contingent imitations of behaviors demonstrated by the child. At this stage the child takes the lead. Recall, prior to 5 to 7 months of age the child will be the primary initiator of communicative interactions, but the adult can keep the interaction going. Contingent imitation has several benefits. First, it allows the child to regulate the amount of social stimulation he or she receives. It also increases the likelihood that adult input will be understood and encourages the child to imitate adult behaviors. This results in the child paying greater attention to the adult and correlates with verbal and vocal performance resulting in greater exploratory play. Finally, it produces more differentiated play activities. These are substantial components of prelinguistic development. In addition, contingent imitation takes advantage of the natural manner in which children show early interest in the world. Also recall that typically developing children, up to approximately 5 to 7 months of age, show initial interest in faces. After that time and following the acquisition of voluntary reach and grasp, children display primary interest in objects. The implication for contingent imitation is obvious. During early stages of prelinguistic intervention, contingent imitation will most likely center on face-to-face interactions between a child and the adult. The child is naturally wired to gaze at faces longer than anything else it may see. Once the child's primary attention shifts to objects, it is logical for contingent imitation activities to switch to objects. Mutual interest in objects of the child's choosing is the cornerstone of reciprocal attention, an important precursor to conversational skills. It is important to mention an additional aspect of children's early communication behavior at this point as well. Up to approximately the age of 5 to 7 months, the child is the primary initiator of communicative interactions, but the adult can prolong the interactions. After that age, the child and the adult can initiate communicative interactions with equal frequency. Once again, the implication for intervention is apparent. What should be communicated to the caregivers (and EI personnel) early is that they should "get their face in the child's face" because this coincides with the child's early and primary interest in faces. Caregivers can be taught how to read a child's early communicative cues. Once adults learn to identify the child's communicative signals, they must be taught how to engage the child in turn-taking activities. Information later in this chapter provides a variety of strategies that the EI can use to alert adults to the type and range of communicative signals a child may send during early stages of prelinguistic development, and how to increase turn-taking behaviors.

An additional approach that may be employed in prelinguistic intervention is an adult's contingent response to a child's current communicative behaviors related to an activity or an object that the child selects or demonstrates interest in. This technique may be referred to as contingent responsivity. The adult's response to child-selected objects or activities facilitates communication development because it enhances and shapes more conventional communicative behavior, which is where the process of prelinguistic development is leading. In essence, this tactic is directing attention toward a child's purposeful (intentional) attentional lead. There are two main reasons why this is superior to attempting to gain the child's attention first and then providing instruction. First, the child's ability to maintain attention toward an adult-selected object is limited. Children are more likely to maintain attention toward an object or activity self-selected by them. Second, the opportunity for contingent responses between the adult and the child is elevated if the contingency is based on a choice expressed by the child.

Building on or adding to (scaffolding) a child's communicative prompts is an additional technique that enhances prelinguistic development. This technique involves giving the child an explicit prompt to imitate a model of a more mature way to communicate a preceding message (Yoder & Warren, 1993). This takes advantage of the child's natural interest in attending to new stimuli when it is incorporated into more familiar stimuli (communicative contexts). This procedure acknowledges that a child is more likely to direct attention toward new words or concepts if they are added to more familiar communicative interchanges and concepts.

Social routines that are a normal part of a child's environment may be incorporated into prelinguistic intervention activities. These routines may be used as a prelinguistic intervention context. The child's early communicative behaviors may be positively influenced and new communicative skills may emerge as predictable patterns of interaction with adults are taken advantage of. Routines may be thought of as repetitive, predictable, turn-taking rituals. These rituals may include games such as peekaboo, patty-cake, and mealtime routines. Many families develop their own simple games (rituals) as part of normal family habits and interactions. The effective EI will inquire about the presence of such routines and assist the adults in using these activities as part of effective prelinguistic intervention. As suggested previously, up to 75% of families of children with special needs never develop such verbal rituals. And yet, it is precisely rituals of this nature that provide the context for turn taking and mutually pleasurable interactions that are the cornerstone for age-appropriate communication development. It is precisely the repetitive and predictable aspect of these behaviors that makes them attractive as an intervention technique. The repetitive structure of these exercises assists children in capturing and remembering appropriate interactive roles with adults and later with other children in play. As rituals of this nature are expanded and the interactive aspects of the roles change due to the adult adding new information, the behaviors remain novel, and the child is more likely to maintain attention. It is suggested that EIs begin keeping a log of suggested verbal rituals that families of children with special needs may employ. For families who have not developed such rituals, the EI can provide suggestions and, if needed, model the appropriate activity.

TOPIC INITIATION AND TOPIC MAINTENANCE

Competent speakers are able to initiate and maintain a topic of conversation. This is a learned skill and the foundation for this ability is established during prelinguistic communication development. A topic may be considered as anything that an adult and child communicate (verbally or nonverbally) about. This is the result of a specific attention-getting activity by one participant in a communicative interchange (Foster, 1985). This definition implies that children are able to initiate topic-related interchanges long before they are able to use language in a sophisticated manner. In essence, they are able to engage in "topics of conversation" through the use of gesture, vocalization, eye gaze, and other nonverbal (prelinguistic) behaviors. Well before a child reaches his or her first birthday, the child is readily able to attract an adult's attention and direct it to an object in the immediate physical environment. In the earliest stages of topic initiation, the target of interest is most likely to be the adult's face, but later this interest changes to objects within sensory contact of the child. By age 2 years, the child is able to use language for the same purpose. The process begins, however, during prelinguistic stages of development.

Topic Initiation

It has been suggested that topic initiation has four basic components (Keenan & Schieffelin, 1976). The first involves the child's ability to attract the attention of the listener. A distinction must be made between a child's purposeful attempts to gain an adult's attention and when an event takes place that results in the child gaining the adult's attention as an incidental behavior. During the earliest stages of prelinguistic development, topic initiation is limited to self-topics. This suggests that the 1-month-old may be able to get the adult's attention, but the attention cannot be directed toward anything other than the child. Adults (caregivers or EI personnel) must acquire the ability to identify and appropriately respond to the child's self-topic communicative initiations. These take varied forms and are frequently missed by the adult.

Topic initiation also involves a second component. This is noted at approximately 5 to 7 months of age when the child achieves the capacity to direct the adult's attention away from oneself and toward an object. As was suggested earlier in this chapter, by 5 to 7 months of age, the child has gained voluntary motor skills enabling it to reach and grasp objects. This newfound ability to grasp and manipulate objects (toys or other familiar objects) is used to attract the adult's attention and interest. Hence, the adult's attention is directed away from the child and to an object. As gestural development takes place, behaviors such as pointing, gazing, and handing objects are noted with increasing frequency. These behaviors are generally established by 12 months of age. The EI must inform adults that the child's primary interest is likely to shift from faces to objects. If this is not done, the adult may assume that the child is no longer interested in topic initiation and misread the child's intentions.

A third component of topic initiation is the child's ability to initiate topics outside of immediate sensory proximity. Thus, abstract or displaced topics may be introduced by the child. This includes a child directing attention toward things that are out of sight, past events, or things generally not part of the here and now (Foster, 1985).

Finally, the child's communicative repertoire expands to include more traditional speech and language behaviors surrounding topics mutually agreed upon regardless of who initiates the turn-taking opportunity. Gesture, vocalizations, and intelligible words may be used to initiate interest in a topic in an attempt to gain the interest and attention of an adult. This constitutes more traditional linguistic expression on the child's part. This final stage is not attained until the precursors (first three components) have been established. The implications for prelinguistic communication intervention are obvious. The child must become a conversationalist, and topic initiation and maintenance are essential if this is to take place.

Topic Maintenance

For topic maintenance to take place, some form of turn taking must emerge. During the process of typical discourse, topics are generally maintained over a sequence of turns. Turn taking becomes essential for topic maintenance. Topic maintenance, like topic initiation, is a learned skill. At 2 years of age, a typically developing child, although limited in speech and language ability, has the skills necessary to demonstrate topic maintenance. This necessitates a supportive communicative partner. The foundational component of caregiver education for infants and toddlers who are communicatively delayed/disordered is to assist the adult in acquiring the ability to identify age-relevant topic initiation attempts, as well as age-relevant topic preservation behaviors on the child's part. As the child's general fund of knowledge about the world increases, topic maintenance expands, resulting in the ability to carry on a dialogue (conversation) at a later point in time. The more turns on a mutually agreed upon topic, the better. Without topic maintenance, turn taking may take place; however, what emerges is a process that may be referred to as a parallel monologue. The adult or child may initiate a conversational exchange, to which the communicative partner responds. However, if an agreed-upon topic is not selected and maintained, each partner carries on a monologue without respect to the topic decided upon by the other. Turn taking may take place; however, true conversation does not. It is surprising to note how frequently adults interact with children and carry on the process (parallel monologue) just described.

REQUESTING AND COMMENTING

Two common behaviors noted in children during pre- and postlinguistic stages of communication development are requesting and commenting. Weatherby et al. (1988) suggest that requesting and commenting are the two most frequent communicative functions expressed during the prelinguistic period. Requesting and commenting provide a framework for contexts in which additional communicative performance is observed. These additional aspects of performance, which descend from requesting and commenting, are intentionality, conventionality, and referencing. Requesting includes behavior that indicates a child wants something and that excludes reflexive activities. Clearly, requesting involves intentionality and conventionality. Referencing may be initially noted in the framework of commenting and is observed when a child is drawing attention to a single object of interest.

In addition to requesting and commenting, children during prelinguistic development display an increased quantity of imitation and participation in social games. These are important components of prelinguistic development and each possesses implications for intervention. It is generally accepted that children learn communication behaviors specific to their language through imitation. Vocal and gestural imitation are both important precursors to language. Imitation may serve the purpose of assisting the child in turn taking when the child does not fully know how to respond. Predictable turn-taking (social) routines are likewise important prelinguistic milestones. Children who are able to demonstrate active participation in social routines are demonstrating greater communicative competence than those who are unable to do so. Table 5–2 presents a summary of communicative functions. The EI may construct intervention activities designed to elicit the communicative functions listed in this table. Two highly practical approaches to understanding communicative functions and from which prelinguistic intervention suggestions flow are provided by McLean and Snyder-McLean (1991) and Weatherby and Prizant (1989). These are summarized in Table 5–3. What these examples imply and what current practice in communication-based intervention symbolizes is that the goal of early intervention is to improve communication skills through a naturalistic and functional (as opposed to form) orientation. Both function and form are necessary for effective communication. However, at the outset functional communication is the goal.

Prelinguistic communication development is a period during which considerable communicative growth takes place. During this period, children gain the ability to intentionally communicate with their world. This all takes place before the child's first words. Gaining this capacity is an important precursor to later linguistic advancement. This early signaling (prelinguistic communication) appears to establish the groundwork for the development of language. The material that follows is intended to provide the EI with a variety of intervention guidelines as well as specific suggestions for communication/language intervention assistance.

SPECIFIC INTERVENTION MODELS, GUIDELINES, GOALS, AND TECHNIQUES

Intervention Models

Behavioral versus Naturalistic Model

Behavioral intervention has been one of the most widely used models for children displaying delayed or disordered communication. The behavioral approach suggests that because language is a learned behavior an adult must elicit and model the correct behavior and appropriately reward the behavior when observed. Thus the child is provided with a stimulus, and the reward response increases the likelihood that the behavior will recur. Once a behavior is repeated,

TABLE 5-2   Communicative Functions

Behavioral Regulation

Request object: Acts used to demand/request a desired object

Request action: Acts used to command another to carry out an action

Protest: Acts used to refuse an undesired object or to command another to cease an undesired action

Social Interaction

Request social routine: Acts used to command another to commence or continue carrying out a gamelike social interaction

Showing off: Acts used to attract another's attention to oneself

Greeting: Acts used to indicate one's notice of another's presence or to signal the termination of an interaction

Calling: Acts used to gain the attention of another, usually to indicate that a communicative act will follow

Acknowledgment: Used to indicate notice of another's previous statement or action; used to indicate a child's focusing attention on or shifting attention to a communicative partner

Request permission: Used to seek another's consent to carry out an action; involves a child carrying out or wanting to carry out an action

Joint Attention

Comment: Acts used to direct another's attention to an entity or event

Request information: Used to seek information

Clarification: Used to clarify a previous utterance

Discourse Structure

Initiated: Child initiates a communication interchange without an adult prompt

Respondent: Child maintains topic through responding

Communicative Means

Gestural: Child uses only his or her body to communicate

Vocal: Child produces an utterance (intelligible or unintelligible)

Verbal: Child uses conventional words

Gestural/vocal: Vocal and gestural behaviors used simultaneously

Gestural/verbal: Gesture and verbal used simultaneously

Adapted from "Analysis of Intentional Communication of Normal Children from the Prelinguistic to the Multiword Stage," by A. Weatherby, D. Cain, D. Yonclas, and V. Walker, 1988, *Journal of Speech and Hearing Research, 31*, p. 240.

TABLE 5–3   Communicative Intent—Functions

From Weatherby and Prizant (1989)

Comment on object:	Acts used to direct another's attention to an entity
Comment on action:	Acts used to direct another's attention to an event
Showing off:	Acts used to attract another's attention to oneself
Calling:	Used to gain the attention of others, usually to indicate that a communicative act is to follow
Acknowledgment:	Used to indicate notice of another person's previous statement or utterance
Clarification:	Used to clarify a previous utterance
Request object:	Used to demand a tangible object
Request action:	Used to command another to carry out an action
Request information:	Used to seek information
Request permission:	Used to seek another's consent
Request social routine:	Used to command another to initiate or continue a gamelike social routine
Protest:	Acts used to refuse an undesired object or to command another to cease an undesired action
Greeting:	Acts used to gain another's attention or indicate notice of another's presence

From McLean and Snyder-McLean (1991)

Request attention:	Used to direct communicative partner's attention to some object, person, or event
Request attention to self:	Used to attract attention to oneself; no other referent is indicated
Request object:	Used to request an object; interest is on the desired object
Request instrumental action:	Used to direct a communicative partner to carry out an action designed to facilitate access to an object or attainment of a desired effect
Request information: feedback:	Used to direct communicative partner to provide information about an object or action
Request noninstrumental action:	Used to direct a communicative partner's actions rather than obtain an object

(continued)

TABLE 5-3 *(continued)*

Request cessation:	Used to request that a communicative partner cease an undesired action or activity

Adapted from "The Expression of Communicative Intent: Assessment Guidelines," by A. Weatherby and B. Prizant, 1989, *Seminars in Speech and Language, 10*, p. 77.

Adapted from "Application of Pragmatics to Severely Mentally Retarded Children and Youth" (p. 50), by J. McLean and L. Snyder-McLean in *Language Perspectives: Acquisition, Retardation, and Intervention*, edited by R. Schiefelbusch and L. Lloyd, 1991, Austin, TX: PRO-ED.

learning is said to have occurred. A behavioral intervention approach suggests that language is learned, and this method affords the child an opportunity to obtain increasingly sophisticated communication skills. As has been previously noted, this model has significant short-comings. Perhaps the biggest shortcoming is a consistent problem with generalization. Children who are communicatively disordered and receive remediation through a behavioral approach to intervention generally fail to transfer newly learned skills to other situations and people (Spradlin & Siegel, 1982). Patrick (1993) has indicated that simple examination of a traditional clinical treatment session designed to improve communication skills readily underscores the limitations inherent in a behavioral approach toward communication intervention. In general, intervention from a behavioral perspective involves one interventionist and one child in a relatively structured setting. The adult predetermines which language structures (forms) are included in the intervention program, as well as the sequence in which they will be learned. The learning that takes place is acquired by the child in a stimulus-response reinforcement paradigm and not within the context of normal discourse. In general, the child may be required to repeat what has been said, name objects and pictures, and describe events or pictures. In such a setting, the child has little control over the interactions or the stimulus materials. The adult chooses the topic of conversation, initiates the turn taking, determines when to switch to a new topic, controls the pace of communication, and generally prefers that the child stick to the preselected topic. In this model the child is generally discouraged from initiating a new topic. In addition, the child has limited opportunity to express individual and/or spontaneous desires, needs, or intentions. In this type of situation, the adult initiates the interaction and maintains control. Instruction is formal, direct, and systematic. This system emphasizes the acquisition of linguistic form and not learning, in general. Children in earlier stages of language development cannot be forced to talk, no matter how skilled the EI. No wonder transfer of learned skills is limited.

The above approach is in sharp contrast to a naturalistic intervention approach. In a naturalistic approach, language is viewed as a process involving a variety of components, not simply language form. A naturalistic approach recognizes that children acquire language through escalating interaction with their environment and through natural conversation. It is characterized as a process that keeps the conversation going. Through this process, children demonstrate a consistent pattern of maturation and growth in their communication skills. A naturalistic approach recognizes that communicative behavior must be established in the context of conversations and interactive routines in a mutually pleasurable manner. It is imperative that children learn to interact in a communicative partnership with a variety of people and in a variety of settings. Conversational exchanges provide multiple opportunities for communication partners to expand a child's overall communication ability. Establishing communicative behavior in a conversational framework affords the greatest opportunity for generalized conversational use. Over time, this strategy enhances the likelihood that a child's utterances and general communicative competencies are expanded and refined, ultimately representing more specific and conventional language performance. As the child's conversational skills improve and as vocabulary growth takes place, the child experiments with more complex grammatical structures in a conversational format. The result is a more natural manner in which increasingly complex language skills are learned, practiced, and incorporated into the child's communicative repertoire.

Play-Based Intervention Model

Play-based intervention is an approach for enhancing communication skills that involves the child in an enjoyable process designed to increase functional language skills. One addition to a play-based approach, particularly for children under 3 years of age, is the involvement of various disciplines, each possessing the ability to cross traditional disciplinary boundaries (role release). This may be referred to as transdisciplinary play-based intervention (Linder, 1993). Transdisciplinary play-based intervention that focuses on enhancing communication skills requires effective dialogue and problem solving among a team of professionals, including parents. The main benefit of this strategy is that it can be readily incorporated into a child's and family's normal routine and may be applied in a home-based or center-based intervention program. It is a flexible process that can follow the child, regardless of primary intervention setting or the professionals involved. It is predicated on several simple principles: (1) children learn best by engaging and interacting with their environment; (2) children learn through social interactions involving communication and problem solving; (3) skills are acquired in increments representing a normal maturational process; (4) play is a significant context in which incremental skills can be learned, practiced, and mastered; (5) one key to development is an adult's encouragement of the child and the degree to which the adult responds to changes in a child's skill level; (6) children learn best through interactions with those most familiar to them and those with whom they feel most comfortable; (7) learning of new skills can be influenced by emotions, both positive and negative; and (8) all aspects of a child's thought (world) are important to functioning. As Linder (1993) suggests, these components contribute to an intervention approach that is child centered, family focused, peer oriented, culturally and developmentally relevant, and based on pleasurable interactions. The approach may be adapted to meet the unique needs of each participant (child and adult) and results in an individualized process geared toward meeting the unique needs of each child in a family-focused context involving various early intervention professionals. Table 5–4 describes the limitations of traditional intervention and the strengths of play-based intervention. These benefits are substantial and lend significant justification to adoption of a transdisciplinary play-based approach to communication-based intervention (Linder, 1993).

Intervention Goals

As has been suggested in the preceding discussion, the overall goal of communication-based intervention is to establish an interactive, communication-based relationship between a child and his or her environment and the adults within the environment. A variety of paradigms can help the EI decide on age-appropriate intervention goals as the process of intervention unfolds. However, regardless of which paradigm (theoretical framework) is adopted, one must keep in mind that the overall intent of all activities is to facilitate a child's ability to interact with his or her world (become a conversationalist). Becoming an interactive communicative partner (conversationalist) on the child's part is the objective. For this objective to be realized, goals

TABLE 5–4 Limitations versus Strengths of Traditional and Play-Based Intervention

Limitations of Traditional (Behavioral) Intervention

Teacher directed: There is limited opportunity for child-directed choice, variety, repetition, and interactions.

Skills driven: Curriculum is driven by weaknesses determined through assessment.

Global goals: Educational approach is characterized by more global intervention goals.

Adult-dominated interactions: Adults provide the bulk of direction and make most choices.

Segregated environment: "Therapy" may be provided in a setting outside of the classroom.

Strengths of Play-Based Intervention

Child-motivated environment: Intervention activities are designed around the child's interests.

Child-directed curriculum: The child's interests dictate the content and direction intervention will take.

Individualized objectives: Objectives are written into the curriculum.

Interaction-focused activities: Relationship with adults is more reciprocal than hierarchical.

Integrated therapy: Skills are acquired and used in a functional format.

Holistic approach: Attention is directed toward the child's abilities in all contexts.

Inclusive classrooms: Children of differing skill levels are included in each classroom.

Adapted from *Transdisciplinary Play-Based Intervention* (p. 210), by T. Linder, 1993, Baltimore: Paul H. Brookes.

must be formulated that take into consideration the adult's role in the intervention process. Information presented later in this chapter elaborates on specific adult goals for the interactive nature of all intervention activities. Additional discussion in this chapter also provides the reader with specific suggestions and techniques to assist in accomplishing the goals discussed here.

The EI must keep both short- and long-term considerations in mind when adopting any system of goals. In other words, the EI must be aware of where the child is initially, where the EI wishes to go next, and what the end product of all intervention activities is to be. Leonard

(1992) has provided early interventionists with several general goals for the development of individualized intervention plans. These goals are discussed, in modified form, in the discussion to follow.

First, intervention should be designed to increase the number of enjoyable and successful communicative interactions the child has with adults. This goal addresses two issues. It reduces the child's potential frustration due to an inability to communicate and it also assists the adult in attaining greater responsivity to the child's communicative behaviors.

A second goal is to increase the child's communicative attempts, with or without prompting. Children who do not demonstrate adequate communicative initiations cannot be effective communicative partners. Communicative success for children who make limited communication attempts is restricted because they do not have ample opportunity to engage in exchanges, verbal or nonverbal, with adults. The EI is encouraged to count and record the manner in which the child initiates conversational exchanges.

Third, it is important that the child learn to respond to adult communication attempts. Again, communication exchanges involve at least two people. The adult must learn to identify the child's communication attempts, just as the child must learn to perceive when the adult is initiating a communicative exchange. Once the child and adult have established more frequent communicative exchanges, it becomes necessary to direct attention toward the intelligibility of a child's utterances. Although this is not a primary goal during the initial stages of intervention, at some time it must be addressed. The child will experience additional frustration if his or her verbalizations are not readily understood by adults or other communicative partners. The goals identified above relate most specifically to communicative behavior.

Information discussed previously in this chapter suggested that intervention activities, although directed toward a specific developmental domain, must be understood in the context of the child's total environment as well as stage of development. Hence, communication-based intervention may incorporate goals that appear more broad in nature. Such is a structure of goals proposed by MacDonald and Carroll (1992). Intervention goals identified in this system include both child and adult goals. The child goals are broken into goals for social play, turn taking, nonverbal communication, language, and conversation. Table 5–5 presents an adapted version of the goals presented by MacDonald and Carroll. As is apparent in the MacDonald and Carroll approach, both prelinguistic and linguistic goals are targeted. This represents a comprehensive and viable way of viewing

TABLE 5–5   Goals for Communication with Infants

Child Goals

Social Play

- Increase interaction
- Preference of social contact to being alone
- Enjoyment of being with people

Nonverbal Communication

- Establish consistent nonverbal communication with others (before language)
- Communicate with movements and sounds
- Communicate back and forth with others
- Respond to others' speech

Turn Taking

- Stay in reciprocal interactions
- Take turns with others
- Share the lead in play
- Imitate others' actions
- Stay in give-and-take exchanges more than briefly

Language

- Express experiences and intentions in words and sentences for communication
- Regularly say new words and combine words into sentences
- Talk about own and others' interests and activities

Conversation

- Stay in balanced conversations for social reasons
- Communicate for friendly contacts
- Take turns in conversations
- Keep the conversation going
- Stay on a topic more than momentarily

Adapted from "A Partnership Model for Communicating with Infants at Risk," by J. MacDonald and J. Carroll, 1992, *Infants and Young Children, 4*, p. 20.

what needs to be accomplished as part of an overall tactic for communication-based intervention. MacDonald and Carroll further suggest that this model adopts the philosophy that children can learn to interact and communicate productively in all instances of interpersonal contact, regardless of the child's communicative status. Thus, all opportunities to interact with the child become opportunities for accomplishing the goals identified in Table 5–5. In essence, this model suggests that children learn best by being proactive rather than reactive in their interactions with adults. The goals specified in Table 5–5 afford the child an opportunity to become a better-equipped proactive communicative partner.

As has been previously noted, prespeech (prelinguistic) skills are paramount for the formation of more traditional language-based behaviors. One system for the establishment of prespeech behaviors is described by Vellman, Davis, and Vihman (1994). In this scheme, several prespeech goals are identified. These prespeech goals are worth noting because they represent a naturalistic approach toward intervention, yet at the same time identify specific intervention goals that may be incorporated into an intervention plan. Prespeech goals, as identified by Vellman, Davis, and Vihman are presented in Table 5–6.

One final approach to establishing communication-based intervention goals is described by Briggs (1992). In the Briggs model, communication-based intervention goals are broken into two main categories, with subheadings under each. A modified version of the Briggs approach is presented in Table 5–7. This is a particularly effective manner of approaching intervention goals because it acknowledges the naturalistic manner in which children acquire communication skills. In addition, it initially emphasizes communicative func-

---

TABLE 5–6   Goals for Prespeech Intervention

Prespeech Continuum Goals

1. *Establish eye contact:* This involves gaining reciprocal attention directed toward one another's faces.

2. *Establish whole body imitation/turn taking:* This involves imitative motor activity, which may include waving bye-bye, throwing a ball, and so on.

3. *Establish fine motor imitation:* This includes imitative behavior by the infant and adult, which may include behaviors such as smiling, kissing, lip movements, sticking out the tongue, and licking.

4. *Increase vocalizations:* Nonmeaningful as well as meaningful vocalizations should be increased and validated when they take place.

5. *Establish consistent pairing of sound and meaning for communication:* This assists the child in transitioning from a prelinguistic to a verbal mode of communication.

Adapted from "Why Do Babies Need Speech Therapy?" Paper presented by S. Vellman, B. Davis, and M. Vihman, 1994, at the annual convention of the American Speech-Language-Hearing Association, San Antonio, TX.

TABLE 5–7   Intervention Goals for Infants and Toddlers

Content-Related Goals

Conversational Routines

Turn taking:	The goal is to increase the child's and adult's understanding of the necessity of turn taking as a conversational strategy.
Initiation:	Both the child and adult must learn to read each other's communicative initiation cues.
Topic maintenance:	It is necessary that the child learn to maintain joint attention in a conversation, regardless of whether the turn taking is verbal or nonverbal.
Termination:	As greater language skills are acquired, the child must learn how to terminate communicative exchanges.

Communicative Functions

Requesting:	The child must learn to use requesting as a strategy for initiating communicative exchanges. This goal may be accomplished through the use of verbal or nonverbal cues.
Denying:	This goal involves the child acquiring more acceptable strategies for denying.
Demanding:	This goal requires the child to demonstrate more acceptable strategies for demanding.
Acknowledging:	As greater language ability is demonstrated, the child will be able to show interest in conversational topics.
Commanding:	Both verbal and nonverbal commanding behaviors make up this goal.
Commenting:	This goal involves the child as an interactive partner who adds to and comments on conversational topics.
Protesting:	Initially, this behavior is nonverbal; however, as an increase in language is noted, intervention will focus on language-oriented protesting behaviors.

Communicative Form

Vocabulary:	As communicative ability increases, an important goal will relate to increasing vocabulary size and content.
Sentence structure:	Communicative form will emerge as an important goal.
Speech intelligibility:	As speech improves, intelligibility of utterances becomes a goal.
Social use:	Pragmatic skills are a later goal of intervention.

Adapted from "Communication Intervention for Infants and Toddlers: A family Context Approach." Paper presented by M. Briggs, 1992, at the annual convention of the Wisconsin Speech-Language-Hearing Association, Oshkosh, WI.

tion, with later emphasis placed on communicative form. The goals contained in the Briggs model are readily modified to fit a play-based naturalistic format of intervention. Additional communication-based intervention goals are presented in Tables 5-8, 5-9, and 5-10.

Regardless of how the EI attempts to define goals, be they short term or long term, global or domain specific, prespeech or language, child initiated or adult initiated, a systematic manner of targeting and moving toward specific communication strategies is paramount. The goals identified in the preceding material are not exhaustive. Rather, the overlap among them is testimony to the universal nature in which

TABLE 5–8   Child Goals to Facilitate Communication

Child Goals

Social Play
- Increase the amount of interaction
- Respond to others with interest
- Prefer social contact to being alone
- Enjoy being in social contexts

Nonverbal Communication
- Establish habitual nonverbal communication patterns with others
- Communicate with movements and sounds
- Communicate back and forth with others
- Respond to others' speech

Turn Taking
- Stay in reciprocal interactions
- Take turns with others
- Share the lead in play
- Imitate others' actions
- Stay in give-and-take exchanges more than briefly

Language
- Express experiences and intentions in words/sentences
- Use new words and word combinations
- Talk about own and others' interests/activities

Conversation
- Stay in balanced conversations for social reasons
- Communicate for friendly contacts
- Take conversational turns
- Keep the conversation going
- Stay on a topic more than momentarily

TABLE 5–9   Adult Goals to Facilitate Communication

Adult Goals

Balance

- Act and communicate as much as child does
- Respond to child's communicative signals
- Initiate communicative exchanges
- Communicate for a response—wait for response
- Sustain joint activities

Responsiveness

- Respond to emerging communication skills
- Respond to child's interests and pace
- Respond to child's actions and communicative signals
- Respond to child's nonverbal communication

Match

- Act and communicate in ways the child can imitate
- Match actions, sounds, words
- Show child how next to communicate
- Be childlike

Nondirectiveness

- Follow the child's lead; allow the child to share in directing the interaction
- Comment more than using questions or commands
- Limit questions to authentic ones

Emotional Attachment

- Become more spontaneously rewarding; engage child more for fun than to get something done
- Actively enjoy the child
- Be animated
- Show childlike play style

those who adopt a naturalistic approach toward communication intervention can move forward. The development of effective communication skills is a maturational process. The goals specified above reflect this and target specific skills designed to accelerate the process.

Intervention Guidelines and Principles

A number of commonsense principles and guidelines must be kept in mind as the EI incorporates specific intervention strategies based on

TABLE 5–10   Age-Related Communication Intervention Goals

Developmental Age	Communication Intervention Goal
0–1 Month	The child will respond reflexively to conversational and environmental sounds.
	The child will arrest activity when a sound is heard.
	The child will be quieted by familiar friendly voices.
	The child's repertoire of responses will be increased to include awareness of new sounds.
1–2 Months	The child will cease activity to attend to unfamiliar voices.
	The child will use body parts to produce sound.
2–3 Months	The child will learn to look directly at the speaker's face.
	The child will associate particular sounds with specific activities.
3–4 Months	The child will learn to turn his or her head deliberately toward the source of sound.
4–5 Months	The child will learn to recognize his or her own name.
	The child will actively make efforts to cause sound to occur through a motor act.
5–7 Months	The child will be made aware of different vocal patterns.
	The child will be able to vocalize to either side.
	The child will attend to music.
	The child will begin to show some understanding of words.
7–10 Months	The child will respond consistently when his or her name is called.
	The child will recognize names of common objects.
	The child will demonstrate some understanding of simple questions.
	The child will cease activity when told "no."
9–12 Months	The child will continue to learn new words.
	The child will localize and fix his or her gaze on a sound source to either side or below the head level.
	The child will listen to speech without being distracted by other sounds.
	The child will follow simple directions with more accuracy than before.
	The child will follow the rhythm of the music.
	The child will understand simple questions.
	The child will respond to rhythmic music with body motion.

Developmental Age	Communication Intervention Goal
	The child will understand an increasing number of verbal requests.
12–16 Months	The child will begin to understand simple categories.
	The child will continue to learn more categories.
	The child demonstrates continued growth in understanding and remembers requests for longer periods of time.
	The child will demonstrate body awareness by identifying basic body parts.
16–20 Months	The child will follow increasingly longer and more difficult directions.
	The child will learn to pick out specified body parts and articles of clothing from pictures upon request.
	The child will learn to discriminate between the pronouns he, she, him, her, I, me, and you.
20–24 Months	The child will follow a series of commands.
	The child will recognize pictures of common objects as well as the objects themselves.
	The child can identify an object from a group of five or more.
24–27 Months	The child will continue to develop understanding of action words.
	The child can identify many more body parts.
	The child will recognize name categories.
27–33 Months	The child will understand the function of objects within general categories.
	The child will begin to understand size differences.
	The child will develop an understanding of descriptive words.
33–36 Months	The child is developing an understanding of prepositions.
	The child will follow directions that are longer and more complex than before.

Adapted from *0–3 Years: An Early Language Curriculum* (p. 50), by C. Reidlich and M. Herzfeld, 1983, Moline, IL: LinguiSystems.

the goals listed. These guidelines have been alluded to in various forms in the material discussed thus far. However, a point-by-point discussion of these principles should serve to assist the EI in implementing the specific intervention strategies in the next section. A brief discussion will follow each principle/guideline. These principles have been gleaned from a vast assortment of sources dealing with communication-based intervention for infants and toddlers.

- *Language emerges from natural conversations and activities that occur between the child and his or her caregivers.* A major premise of this chapter and the entire text is that effective communication skills are not learned in a clinic or laboratory, but rather through natural interactions between the child and his or her world. As such, the intervention strategies that the EI employs should take advantage of naturally occurring events in a child's world to enhance communication and language learning. The EI should not feel the need to manufacture settings in which language might take place. Child-directed activities serve to maintain the child's interest, as well as increase the likelihood that newly learned skills will generalize to other settings. Adult-manufactured conversational opportunities need not be viewed as the goal. Rather, conversational exchanges and opportunities that emerge as part of routine daily caregiving activities should be stressed. Parents engage in a number of daily activities that are rich sources of conversational turn taking. Activities such as mealtime, bathing, dressing, feeding, bedtime, and free play make up the type of activities that are suggested here. Verbal rituals that emerge as part of the typical caregiving routine should be identified and encouraged. It is precisely rituals of this nature that are most naturalistic, rewarding, pleasurable, and beneficial for effective communication partnering to take place. For children with special needs, the EI may need to teach the caregiver how to initiate such rituals and demonstrate their interactive nature.

- *Intervention must involve both the child and his or her caregivers.* Significant attention has been directed thus far to the premise that the child is no longer the main focus of intervention. Rather, the family becomes the focus of all intervention activities. In most instances, the family is the constant in the child's life. From an efficacy standpoint, those children whose caregivers are involved demonstrate more progress in communication skills than those whose caregivers are not involved. It is simply not possible to incorporate a conversational approach toward communication-based intervention apart from caregiver participation. This is one of the main benefits of home-based early intervention. Hence, the EI must direct significant attention toward facilitating the primary caregiver's involvement in communication-based intervention. Caregivers must be shown that their involvement is needed, pleasurable for the adult and child, and will result in greater progress than if they are not involved. Caregiver involvement in all aspects of intervention planning and implementation is not an option but an integral part of the process.

- *Turn taking becomes a critical skill and tool for natural language teaching.* To keep the conversation going, both the child and adult must acquire the ability to send and interpret meaningful communicative signals, verbal or nonverbal. Without this ability, neither communicative partner is able to respond in a manner for conversation to continue. We do not communicate effectively using one word. Nor can communication skills develop if only one turn is allowed in a conversational exchange. Hence, turn taking is a critical skill that must be encouraged, taught, and rewarded for all communicative partners. As mentioned previously, at the outset the best measure of communication progress is not the number of words used by the child but the number of communication initiations the child makes and the number of turns on a single topic. Overriding all communication-based intervention is the premise that turn taking is at the heart of becoming a conversational partner.
- *Nearly all children who are communication/language delayed offer nonlinguistic acts that are infrequently and inappropriately responded to by adults.* Many caregivers falsely assume that their child, due to the degree of disability the child possesses or the child's age, is unable to send or respond to communicative signals. One of the more important messages to convey to caregivers is that the opposite is true. Nearly all children, regardless of degree of deficit, are able to send and respond to communicative initiations and signs. These initiations may be infrequent, nontraditional, fleeting, or otherwise hard to identity. However, the central idea that must be conveyed is that these communicative signals do take place and that the caregiver may need assistance in identifying them. Many caregivers expect the typical "Gerber baby" style of interaction. This is not the case for many children described in the preceding chapters. This is a crucial concept to convey because many parents will devote significant early effort in an attempt to engage the child in interactions. In the

absence of expected responses by the child, the adult may become discouraged and cease communicative exchanges. This is a mistake. The EI must be alert to the potential that the caregiver may become discouraged if typical child responses are not forthcoming. Once parents stop such attempts, it may be difficult to get them to try again. This is a situation in which the EI must be aware of caregiver attempts (successes and failures) early in the intervention process. In those instances when the primary caregiver is slow or reluctant to develop turn-taking skills, the EI is encouraged to look for someone else in the child's immediate caretaking environment who may more readily participate in turn-taking exchanges with the child. The EI should never assume who the good turn taker may be. It may not be the primary caregiver but a secondary member of the family or a member of the extended family. It should also be recalled that turn taking can be taught, and for some parents added instruction and modeling is needed. Perhaps a sibling, grandparent, or member of the extended family may be engaged in these activities if the primary caregiver is reluctant or needs additional time to learn these skills.

- *Adults/caregivers must be taught how to respond in ways that will ultimately enhance and increase more conventional language responses on a child's part.* Information presented in earlier chapters suggested that parents very highly rate their need for accurate information about the specific issues, medical and otherwise, surrounding their child. This is particularly true regarding adult interaction with children displaying delayed communication. Adults can learn effective communicative strategies with such children. However, this does not take place spontaneously. Hence, intervention geared to the child must, of necessity, involve a significant amount of adult-oriented suggestions for improving communicative interactions between adult and child. As a general rule, the younger the child, the more the emphasis on the caregiver and providing them with needed information. As the child gets older, the point is reached at which increasing intervention activity is child centered. More specific information on this is presented later in this chapter.

- *The goal of intervention activities is not to finish the planned activity, but rather to stimulate and elicit communication.* Many interventionists believe that the amount of "talking" a child does is the best measure of their effectiveness. In addition, adults (caregivers) may question the goals of communication-based intervention if the EI is not attempting to achieve verbal output (words) by the child. What must be accepted is that the initial goals of communication-based intervention are to identify a child's learning and interactive style, as well as to identify spontaneous instances in which communication can be stimulated. The overall goal in an individual treatment session is not to finish a planned activity, but rather to elicit communicative behavior. The behavioral approach toward intervention, previously discussed, stressed the completion of specific language-oriented goals (measurable and readily identified). Although setting goals is an important part of intervention, the primary purpose is not to finish a planned activity as the next step toward a preset goal. Rather, the primary purpose is to gain the child as a communicative partner. The EI is encouraged to identify those times when the child sends communicative signals indicative of interest outside of planned activities by the interventionist. This takes maturity and confidence on the part of the clinician. It involves the EI's ability to follow the child's lead and flow with the child's communication initiations, even if they fall outside of what the EI intended.

- *Arrange the environment and activities to enhance potential for communicative interactions.* Children learn most effectively when the EI is aware of and incorporates effective developmental stages into treatment. Recall that children are primarily interested in faces. After voluntary reach and grasp is established, children shift their primary attention toward objects. It is precisely information of this nature that the EI must become familiar with. Developmentally appropriate intervention activities are essential if maximal effectiveness is to be achieved. There is a significant advantage to home-based intervention for this very reason. Toys, setting, and people are quite familiar to the child in the context of the home.
- *Do not try to force verbal output.* As has been suggested, the best measure, particularly early in the intervention process, is not the number of words the child uses. Parents may ask the EI to more fully explain the goals that are targeted as part of the intervention process. In other words, after a while the parent may question why the EI engages the child in play, seemingly random in nature, rather than require the child to use words to express herself. It is not uncommon to hear par-

ents say, "You have been playing with my child for some time now; when will Bobbie start talking?" It must be explained to parents that communication skills (initiation and turn taking) precede talking. These skills are centered upon communication initiations and turn taking.

- *A variety of communication/language-eliciting techniques must be employed.* The overall goal of communication-based intervention is to keep the conversation going. In that context, a variety of strategies may be employed. These include imitation, modeling, questioning, paraphrasing, language expansion, and sentence completion activities. The overall goal is to promote spontaneous communication skills in naturalistic, ongoing exchanges. This process takes time and the EI must first self-cultivate personal skills in employing these strategies. Chaining is a most effective technique when engaging the child in turn-taking activities. Chaining involves the adult adding information to the child's utterance, for the purpose of the child adding even more information of explanation.

- *Learn to use periods of silence during communicative exchanges.* Many EIs believe that periods of silence during intervention must be avoided. Hence, what would be silent periods are filled with talking. Rich communicative exchanges can take place in the absence of talking. In many instances, silence is followed by increased communicative attempts by a child. It should be noted that nonverbal communication can take place during any intervention session, and these periods of communication (nonverbal/silent) should not be avoided if they are part of a larger attempt to enhance communicative exchanges. If the EI bombards the child with verbalizations during treatment, the child may be overwhelmed and reluctant to initiate turn-taking opportunities. Silence should not be feared or viewed as negative in the context of eliciting conversational exchanges.

- *Action-oriented activities stimulate communicative exchanges to a greater degree than pictures.* For children under 3 years of age, there appears to be something essential about action. In essence, children tend to learn best through action, not pictures. The EI is encouraged to incorporate intervention techniques that are action oriented. The use of pictures may tend to stimulate only one-word responses. Children are not effective communicative partners if their utterances consist of one-word responses. Action-oriented activities in spontaneous play-based contexts tend to facilitate increased turn taking for children. In general, it is suggested that the EI avoid pictures, at least until the child becomes an effective communicative partner and is able to maintain a topic for five to seven turns. Then pictures may be used to strengthen vocabulary skills, introduce new concepts, and so on.

- *Be alert to opportunities to expand newly learned communication skills to other settings and contexts.* The principle inherent in this goal is that of generalization. Once a child begins to use more turn taking, it is imperative that other adults in the child's caregiving routine be informed of the progress the child is showing. Clinicians frequently report that generalization is the aspect of intervention with which they struggle most. The EI is strongly encouraged to keep adults informed of progress and specific aspects of a child's communicative skills in an effort to increase the child's use of newly learned communicative abilities in various environmental settings. Asking the parents to keep a communication log is most helpful in this regard. If parents are given a specific assignment (monitoring and recording communication changes), they will be more likely to be aware of progress as it takes place.

- *Avoid yes/no questions as much as possible.* Perhaps the quickest way to end turn-taking exchanges is to structure interactions around yes/no questions. Most adults tend to initiate communication exchanges with children through the use of yes/no questions. It is simple, direct, and adult initiated and directed, yet it is the death of communication exchanges (turn taking). If the child responds with a yes/no answer, the opportunity for turn taking is restricted. What the adult generally does is ask another yes/no question, thus perpetuating one-word responses that do not give the child a chance to initiate or add information. This is an important principle to keep in mind. EI professionals are encouraged to develop a storehouse of techniques that engage children in turn taking apart from reliance on yes/no questions. This is something that must be consciously worked on by the EI. A variety of techniques may serve to better initiate conversations. Lead-in phrases such as "Tell me about. . ." or "How can we..." are preferable. Better yet, the EI is encouraged to simply engage in a play routine while looking for opportunities to participate in turn-taking routines, both verbal and nonverbal. This affords a more naturalistic manner of entering conversational opportunities with the child and proves less threatening, particularly if parents or previous teachers have tried to force verbal output on the child.

● *Primary attention should be directed toward functional communication skills and not language structure.* At the outset of intervention, the overall goal should be to facilitate functional communication skills, with minimal emphasis placed on structural accuracy. This is not meant to minimize the importance of language structure. However, for many children receiving communication-based intervention, any type of communication (especially functional communication) is paramount. Later in the intervention process, increased attention may be directed toward structurally accurate communication.

An example can underscore this concept, as well as point out a corollary principle. It is generally accepted that mothers demonstrate more interest in language structure than fathers. Further, it is likewise accepted that fathers are more interested in functional accuracy (informational content) than mothers. Take, for example, the 5-year-old child who runs quite excitedly into the home and announces, "I runded around the yard 10 times." How might each parent respond? The mother (primary interest in language structure) is likely to respond by saying, "No, honey, you didn't runded around the yard 10 times, you ran around the yard 10 times. You ran around the yard." Dad, on the other hand (primary interest in content accuracy), is more likely to respond by saying, "Come on, I saw you. You only runded around the yard 3 times."

Which communicative partner is correct, Mom or Dad? At the outset, the primary goal is functional communication, perhaps at the expense of structural integrity. Later in the intervention process, increased attention may be directed toward language structure.

DEVELOPMENTAL READINESS STAGES

An additional element is important to mention at this point. How should the EI respond when a child begins to demonstrate rapid progress as a result of the intervention provided? Initially, the clinician may tend to feel quite good and rightfully so. At times, progress is slow and when it does take place, caregivers and clinicians should feel some degree of satisfaction. However, an important concept should be kept in mind. Some clinicians, when rapid progress takes place, may have a natural tendency to "pour it on." That is to say, many EIs become accustomed to slow progress and, in the presence of rapid progress, naturally may tend to become excited. This may translate into attempts to maximize the growth spurt that the child is demonstrating. Yet, the concept of developmental readiness stages must be recalled.

The human development literature has for some time discussed the concept of "developmental readiness stages." It is not a difficult principle to understand. A developmental readiness stage is just what the phrase implies. It represents a time in the developmental sequence when a child is uniquely ready to learn a new skill. It is a time when all precursors to learning a particular skill are completed and the new skill emerges, perhaps quite suddenly. There is very little the EI can do to facilitate the onset or occurrence of a developmental readiness stage. The basic rule is that the readiness stage will take place when the child is ready and not before.

However, is it possible that a developmental readiness stage (growth spurt) can be shortened by events other than health issues? The answer to this question is yes. It is possible for a child to become satiated with intervention activities—satiated to the point at which the child no longer benefits from the intervention. In fact, ongoing intervention (pouring it on) may be counterproductive. In a previous discussion of infant states (Chapter 3), the point was made that infants in the intensive care nursery may exhibit a state referred to as the in-turned state. Recall that this is a state when the child is overloaded by health and environmental influences. The child shuts out the world and any attempts the world makes to interact. The child is overloaded. Clinicians can attempt to reduce the overload effect of the environment but can do little else to shorten the in-turned state.

An important principle previously mentioned should be reinforced. The point was made that EI professionals are simply substitutes for nature. As such it must be recalled that no matter how competent an EI may be, we will never beat nature. At the most, all that can be hoped for is that effective intervention will function as a substitute for nature. The point to be made is obvious. When a child enters a growth spurt, one possible course of action for the EI is to dismiss the child from intervention for a period of time and let nature take its course. At the very least, the clinician should consider a reduction in treatment to avoid satiation of the child. This is not to suggest that the EI lose touch with the child and caregivers. This is a perfect time to encourage the primary caregiver to keep a detailed developmental log of progress noted. It is also suggested that the EI maintain regular contact with the caregivers to more fully monitor the growth taking place. Communication with caregivers is essential during such a time. Once the EI suspects that the growth spurt is slowing or that the child would benefit from reenrollment in more formal intervention, intervention services can be reinstated. Although this may be an unfamiliar concept for many clinicians, experienced early intervention professionals have come to appreciate the need to monitor the intensity of services in light of rapid developmental change.

INTERVENTION TECHNIQUES

The overall intent of communication-based intervention is to facilitate communication development, mirroring the natural way in which language emerges in the context of conversational strategies. The material that follows is designed to assist the clinician in structuring a sequential approach toward intervention, as well as to suggest specific intervention techniques. EI professionals are encouraged to expand their "bag of tricks" in arriving at applicable intervention procedures.

Although the following material is not exhaustive, it should serve to assist the clinician in arriving at effective communication-based intervention activities. A sequential, stage-by-stage approach toward intervention is suggested. No specific ages are attached to each stage. Rather, the stages represent communication skill level rather than chronological age. It is recommended that a child achieve mastery within a stage before the clinician moves on to the next stage. No timetable for mastery within each stage is suggested. The recommended activities within each stage are provided as commonsense intervention recommendations.

As Leonard has noted, four underlying philosophical points underscore communication-based intervention (Leonard, 1992). The first is the application of a developmentally appropriate practice. This suggests that one considers a child's developmental status when beginning intervention. Although chronological age is important as intervention is structured, chronological age is not paramount. Rather, the child's communicative ability (stage) at a given time must be acknowledged. This requires an awareness of the child's skill level as well as learning style. The second point of emphasis covers family involvement in all aspects of intervention. Regardless of treatment strategies employed, individual child goals, materials and curricula used, or setting of intervention, the family is an integral part of the process. As a result, parental resources, priorities, and situation become driving forces in determining the course that intervention will take. Third, care must be taken to match, as best as possible, the adopted intervention strategies and approaches with the individual characteristics of each child and family. This results in more focused intervention and facilitates the development of skills while maximizing family resources. Finally, the issue of flexibility must be kept in mind. Needs of a child and family may change markedly, perhaps without warning. The interventionist cannot become locked into one approach and ignore changes that take place. Ongoing reanalysis of the effectiveness of intervention is paramount. The interventionist must be willing and able to change course on short notice when the need to do so becomes apparent.

Phase I: General Readiness

The readiness phase is the earliest stage of communication development/intervention. This is a time when a child's earliest communication skills are established. It is characterized primarily by a child's initial interest in faces and things. The child's primary activity is gazing or directing visual attention toward people or objects. Of primary concern for many children in this stage are issues related to positioning. For a child to benefit from adult communicative attempts, gazing, visual attention, and reduction of distance become important. In essence, the clinician becomes aware that babies with motor difficulties may require special care when being handled for normal caregiving as well as for intervention purposes. Being aware of how a child is positioned during intervention activities and play is important in setting up the best context for language learning. For the sick or fragile child, proper positioning may be needed to facilitate adequate respiration, head support, trunk support, or general ability to direct attention toward a desired object. Parents and professionals may become frustrated when attempts to direct the child's attention are not successful, only to find out that the child's position was inadequate and at the heart of the difficulty. Although a complete discussion of positioning is outside the scope of this chapter, a basic understanding of positioning issues and suggestions follows.

Children generally need several basic movement abilities to optimally interact with their world. As they grow, infants learn to control and adjust their heads to line up with the middle of their bodies. Even adults, when shifting position or during most motor acts, generally and unconsciously adjust head position to line up with the spine. Infants with motor difficulties may lack the ability to do this; thus, they cannot firmly maintain head support or readily turn their head to explore the environment. This makes it difficult for the child to initiate, maintain, and engage in eye contact with adults. Establishing and maintaining eye contact is a very important part of language learning. A child must be able to maintain attention (initially visual attention) to people and things. Initially, attention is directed toward watching the caregiver's face and facial expressions and later toward looking at mobiles and toys (objects). In an earlier discussion, it was noted that typically developing children up to 5 to 7 months of age are primarily interested in faces, but after that time primary interest shifts to objects. Thus, eye contact with faces and objects is an essential aspect of communication development. In addition, many clinicians provide services for children with visual problems. In instances in which a child's visual skills are impaired, the infant's attention must be shifted from visual stimuli to auditory and tactile stimuli.

An infant who is approaching independent sitting must have adequate trunk support. Low muscle tone (floppy) or a stiffened and extended posture (high tone) can interfere with good interaction patterns. The EI must direct attention toward trunk support during the earliest stages of communication-based intervention. In addition, adequate breath support for later developing speech is essential. One byproduct of monitoring trunk support is maximizing the probability that adequate breath support for speech will develop. For maximal learning (gazing and visual attention) to take place, the child must be in a supported and comfortable position. If a floppy baby is held with inadequate support, the infant will direct energy toward trying to stabilize and support his or her body. As a result, the child cannot become an active participant in play. Infants who receive adequate support and are comfortably positioned will be able to focus greater attention on interactive partners and objects. They will not have to work as hard to maintain body support. Table 5–11 presents some elementary positioning suggestions for children that will facilitate attention and interaction. These suggestions are designed to assist the child in achieving necessary precursors to later communication development.

Phase II: Reciprocity

As has been previously noted, turn taking becomes the centerpiece for language learning. Turn taking begins with the establishment of reciprocal actions between the child and caregivers. Turn taking may be established in several ways. Certainly one technique involves the

TABLE 5-11 Positioning Suggestions

Child in Parent's Arms

- Cradling a child in the arms during feeding provides good support for the child along the entire length of the child's body.
- For an older child, a pillow may be used to prop up the child while on the parent's lap. The pillow will assist the child in maintaining an upright position and facilitate good eye contact. The chin should be held with one hand, if head support is inadequate.

Child Lying on Back

- Place a small pillow or folded towel under the child's shoulders and head. This is helpful for the child who tends to overextend the body.
- Sit on the floor with your back to the wall and cradle the child in your lap facing you. The child's body will conform to the contour of your lap.

Child Lying on Tummy

- Provide a large pillow support under the child's body. Place a colorful toy or mirror 8 to 10 in. from the child's face.
- For an older child, place a smaller pillow or wedge under the child's chest. Provide a toy (to encourage reaching) or a mirror to play with.
- Lie on the floor with a pillow under your head and the child lying on your stomach. Support the child's shoulders. A child with adequate head support will be able to look directly at you.

Child Sitting (once child is ready for upright sitting)

- Have the child sit on your abdomen facing you, and provide support at the elbows and forearms.
- Have child sit with knees bent and soles of feet touching, forming a ring. The child may also extend one leg in a half-ring sit.

Adapted from *Growing Together: Communication Activities for Infants and Toddlers* (p. 200), by M. Devine, 1990, Tucson, AZ: Communication Skill Builders.

use of social (ritual) games. Activities such as peekaboo, patty-cake, and "how big is baby" lend themselves to joint attention (adult and child) and reciprocal interaction. The EI is encouraged to assist families in identifying and expanding any natural games that have spontaneously developed as part of the normal caregiving routine. The clinician must become aware of instances when the child's visual attention can be directed toward a mutual point of interest. Although visual attention is initially directed to faces, it will shift to objects, particularly after the child establishes voluntary reach and grasp. Feeding routines, breast or bottle, can serve as a primary point of joint attention (face to face). Caregivers routinely report how quickly the child becomes aware of signals sent by the adult that signify feeding time is approaching. A simple act, such as unzipping a diaper bag to retrieve a bottle, can direct a child's attention toward feeding activity. As the length of a child's attention span increases, toys and everyday objects may be used to expand the repertoire of things the child demonstrates interest in. It is imperative that the adult be alert to the range of articles toward which a child will voluntarily direct attention. Likewise, the adult must become aware of any objects in the child's environment (usually as part of normal caregiving) that the child's attention may be directed toward. The adult should be alert to the variety of ways the child indicates that he or she has directed attention toward something. Once the child's interest is detected by the adult, mutual interest should be pursued for as long as the child maintains interest.

These first two phases of intervention are designed primarily to increase the number of enjoyable and successful communicative opportunities that take place between the child and adult. Further, they alert the adult to the natural manner in which communication interactions take place. This is a time during which the adult's responsivity to the child's interest (attention) may be heightened. This is an important step and must not be shortened or minimized. The result is that communicative routines are established in which the child may participate. Readiness and joint attention serve to alert the adult to the child's nonverbal cues. The adult is then encouraged to respond to the child's (prelinguistic) signals as if the child had communicated verbally. As a result, the child is rewarded for communicative signals, thereby increasing their frequency.

Medically fragile children engaged in phase I or phase II intervention activities will generally demonstrate responsivity to signals, as well as send communicative signals. However, these are more subtle in nature and more difficult to detect. Clinicians and parents must take the time to identify a child's communicative initiations and responses, regardless of the setting. All children send some type of communicative signal, however frequently missed by adults. Previous information suggested that caregivers will generally devote a tremendous amount of time attempting to engage their child in interactions. However, if an adult receives no feedback for these efforts, the attempts become less frequent and eventually may cease. This must be avoided if at all possible. Once the efforts cease, the adult may be reluctant to try again. Hence, the clinician must help the caregiver identify communicative signals and responses a child may display. Cessation or lessening of motor activity, changes in breathing, changes in skin color (for hospitalized infants), widening of the eyes, rhythmic motor movements accompanying speech, and attempts to find and identify a communicative partner are all signals that a child is aware of an adult's presence.

Phase III: Social-Communicative Signals

Once a child has moved through the two previous stages and is demonstrating consistent attention toward people and objects, the focus of intervention changes to include increased socio-communicative content. This is a time when vocalic, motoric, and gestural actions are linked. It is a time during which contingent relationships between gesture, motor movements, and vocalizations are stressed. The adult must be aware of the manner in which a child links vocalizations, motor activity, and environmental experiences to signify the child's intentional communication. At first these linkages may be quite subtle and fleeting. Later, as the child gains confidence in the ability to attract and maintain adult attention, the length and complexity of these interactions will increase. It is during this phase that the adult may use frequent repetitions of the child's vocalizations, as well as introduce words and short phrases to describe the activity that the child draws attention to, *not forcing verbal output*. The adult is encouraged, during this phase, to dramatically vary vocal intonation and intensity. This focuses the child's attention and increases the likelihood of imitative attempts on the child's part. Messages sent by the adult should be accompanied by gesture, heightened facial expression, and body language. The adult speaking rate should be slowed, clearly articulated, and reflect a reduced length of utterance (four to seven words). Frequent repetition of verbalizations (by the adult), repetitive introduction of objects and actions, and pleasurable and animated exchanges are encouraged.

Phase IV: Early Language Comprehension

Once the child is demonstrating increased attention toward language and increased vocalizations (perhaps unintelligible), the focus shifts to activities designed to increase language comprehension. This is a subtle shift and may be evidenced by the child demonstrating enhanced awareness of objects or people when named. The child may express consistent preference for certain activities or objects, further indicating an increased comprehension ability.

A variety of play-oriented activities may be introduced to assist in maintaining and expanding a child's interest in vocalizations. These may include finger activities, sound play, telephone play, and specific play routines tied to objects of the child's choosing, as well as other play activities. During this phase, the adult may consistently label items in the child's environment. If a child begins to use a word meaningfully, frequent reward and reinforcement should take place. Modeling may be consistently used. The adult may "coach" the child to imitate a word that reflects an object or activity with which the child has demonstrated familiarity. The child may be encouraged to look at objects when named, identify body parts, identify family members, point to familiar toys, display motor movements reflective of words, or generally demonstrate increased awareness and accuracy in signifying increased language comprehension. Table 5–12 presents additional activities and suggestions that fit into this phase of intervention. During previous intervention activities, liberal use of gesture on the part of the adult was suggested. The clinician, when measuring or monitoring language comprehension skills, must be careful to use gesture in a manner that does not confound attempts to gauge lan-

TABLE 5–12   Sample Activities to Enhance Language Comprehension

Cooperates in games: The child enjoys the give-and-take of simple games. The child understands the routine of the game and vocalizes as part of the game activity.

Shows like/dislike for people and objects: The child demonstrates definite likes and dislikes for people, objects, or games. If the name of the object, person, or activity is provided, the child protests.

Extends toy when named by adult: The child extends an object when the object is named by the adult.

Begins to show sense of humor: The child laughs when an activity is described, imitated, or recalled.

Child demonstrates gesture on request: Child blows kisses, waves bye-bye, or imitates other motor activities when requested by adult.

Child understands "no": The child may shake head or in another manner indicate the concept of "no."

Child sorts objects: When requested by an adult, the child is able to sort objects.

Gives one out of many: The child gives or takes one of something from a larger grouping, free from unintentional cuing.

guage comprehension apart from gesture. Gesture should still be used by the adult; however, increased reliance on verbal cues alone is the target at this stage.

Phase V: Language Expression

The final phase of communication-based intervention is one in which the emphasis shifts to language expression by the child. This is a time when an adult must be alert to and enhance all vocalization attempts. This includes both intelligible and unintelligible utterances, particularly if intentional in nature. A variety of activities may be included during this phase of intervention. Table 5–13 presents some suggested language expression activities. One common technique that may prove useful during this stage of intervention is expansion. Expansion is an adult response that involves repeating the child's utterance and adding one or two additional and appropriate features. Word production is worked on liberally with consistent regard for word usage. Attention is directed toward linking objects and activities with words, while at the same time attempting to expand the mean length of each

TABLE 5–13   Suggested Language Expression Activities

Experiments with communication: The child may be encouraged to play with words. The adult may encourage the production of new sounds, words, and perhaps, short phrases in an attempt to expand language expression.

Single-word sentences: As the child begins to display single-word production, caregivers reward and expand on the child's utterances.

Greetings: The child is encouraged to say "hi" and "bye" with and without gesture.

Naming familiar objects: The child is encouraged to provide appropriate names for familiar objects or activities.

Singing: The child is expected to sing along with familiar songs.

Imitates noises: The child is exposed to environmental noises and animal noises and asked to imitate them.

Answers questions: When presented with simple questions, the child is expected to provide appropriate answers (short answers).

Nursery rhymes: The child is assisted in learning nursery rhymes and is encouraged and praised for saying them.

utterance the child offers. The clinician must not lose sight of the overall objective, which is to increase turn taking between communicative partners. Hence, it is preferable that the child frequently initiate communicative interchanges and take adequate turns rather than be able to name or identify multiple objects outside a conversational (turn taking) context. Leonard (1992) has provided a helpful outline of activities that may be used with children to enhance communicative abilities as the child progresses through the phases identified in this section. These activities are presented in modified form in Table 5–14.

Transition from phase to phase is generally not dramatic, but rather slow and sometimes quite subtle. There is no clear line that separates each phase. Rather, the skills described in each phase should be thought of as a continuum from the earliest of communicative opportunities to later full participation in communicative interchanges by the child. Accurate record keeping, the use of a parental log, videotaping, and alerting the parents to all aspects of communication skills as they emerge will enhance intervention effectiveness overall.

As the child's skills increase and more complex language structures and activities are incorporated into intervention, several additional principles must be recalled. Intervention for children displaying increased language usage may focus on four basic components. First, attention may be directed toward general concepts. This can include concepts such as size, shapes, colors, categorization, and so on. The goal of incorporating concept expansion into intervention is to boost the child's ability to generalize newly learned language skills to other environmental and conversational situations. Generalization of newly learned skills continues to be one of the interventionist's most frequently reported frustrations. One way to enhance generalization is to expand as many concepts as possible. This is dictated by the child's level of mastery and interests. A second feature that must be stressed in later stages of intervention are vocabulary skills. The child may be exposed on a regular basis to new vocabulary items. These may be new items in the child's immediate environment or other vocabulary items the child shows interest in. Caregivers should be instructed to keep a record of the child's areas of interest. The EI may capitalize on these areas of interest in expanding the child's overall vocabulary size. Third, the point is reached when functional communication is progressing nicely and attention must be directed toward language structure. Through the conversational strategies (modeling, expansion, coaching, paraphrase), the child can be exposed to appropriate language structures. As this ability increases,

TABLE 5–14 Communication Intervention Techniques

Input Strategies

- Slow speech rate. Speak in a slow, clear manner.
- Converse face to face. Sit so that you are face to face with the child.
- Shorten the length of your typical utterance. Use utterances that resemble the length of the child's utterances.
- Use frequent repetition.
- Consistently label items familiar to the child. Once comprehension is attained, generalize the item named to various contexts.
- Use variety in vocal intensity and intonational patterns.
- Use parallel talk. Describe your ongoing activities and interests.
- Use self-talk, which describes your ongoing activities.
- Use frequent modeling. Say words and phrases that are related/cued to the immediate context.
- Coach the child to use a word or phrase at the appropriate time and situation.
- Provide answers and conversation at the child's utterance level.

Responsive Strategies

- Use frequent repetitions of the child's utterances.
- Expand on the child's utterances. Repeat the child's utterances, adding additional features.
- Repeat elements of the child's utterance, slightly changing the initial construction (paraphrase).
- If needed, provide words to express the child's feelings. Provide words to assist the child in expressing feelings when the child is unable to do so.
- Reward and highlight words and phrases that are emerging in the child's expressive repertoire.
- Change immature utterances to more mature and recognizable ones.

Clarification Strategies

- Repeat any part of the child's utterance that is understood.
- When the child's intended meaning is unclear, ask choice questions to clarify the meaning.
- Ask the child to show you what he or she means when utterances are not understood.
- Be alert to topics that the child frequently talks about. Contextual information may increase adult listening ability.
- If the child is not understood, the adult may choose to take responsibility.

Adapted from "Communication Intervention with Young Children at Risk for Specific Communication Delay," by L. Leonard, 1992, *Seminars in Speech and Language, 13*, p. 223.

both language function and form more closely mirror age-appropriate communication skills.

A final area that can receive attention during language intervention is language usage (pragmatics). Specific conversational situations can be presented in a play context that assist a child in acquiring age-appropriate and socially acceptable rules for language usage. During the later aspects of intervention, the EI needs to be aware of issues relating to behavioral control, control of stimulus materials, maintaining the child's interest and enthusiasm, and using interesting materials and activities.

The overall premise of the presented intervention suggestions is that the EI represents a substitute for nature and, as such, a naturalistic model of intervention must be employed. A variety of common-sense suggestions for structuring intervention, as well as specific intervention activities, have been presented. The entire early intervention team, regardless of primary academic disciplines, will benefit from the suggestions offered.

TRAINING PARENTS AS COMMUNICATION/LANGUAGE FACILITATORS

In the material presented thus far, consistent mention has been made of the parents' role in early intervention. In fact, most textbooks that provide suggestions about effective communication intervention make specific mention of the importance of training parents and significant others as language facilitators. In a 1979 study conducted by Cartright and Ruscello, approximately 89% of respondents (early intervention facilities) to a national survey indicated that their facility viewed parent involvement as an essential component of clinical services. However, only 51% of those who considered parent involvement to be essential indicated that their centers had actually organized such programs. Of those who indicated that parent involvement was established, 62% indicated that the approach most frequently used was to develop printed materials for distribution to parents. The role parents play in intervention and subsequent efficacy is perhaps most apparent in the development of communication skills. Early intervention professionals must develop effective strategies designed to engage parents in the process and, more specifically, to help them become effective communication facilitators. A child's earliest model will be the primary caregiver. Hence, anything the EI can do to improve caregiver understanding of the importance of effective communication skills will improve overall child outcome.

Two questions emerge about caregiver involvement in communication facilitation. First, does it work? In other words, can parents be effectively taught how to improve their interactive skills with children? The answer to this first question is yes. A complete discussion of the efficacy of training parents as communication facilitators is presented in Chapter 6. The second question relates to how EI professionals can train parents to become effective communicative partners for their children at risk for communication delay. What specific skills are needed? Are there materials designed to assist parents in becoming effective communicative partners?

Parent Training

One approach in training parents as language facilitators is presented by McDade and Varnedoe (1987). This approach reflects a view that parents are not to take the place of the clinician, but rather that parents are trained to function as general language facilitators. As McDade and Varnedoe suggest, two basic approaches are available to EI personnel in attempting to structure adults' interactions with children displaying communication delay. First, adults can be taught the skills necessary for maintaining a child's attention so that it may be directed toward specific items and activities. This approach may tend to be more adult directed (trainer oriented). In the trainer-oriented approach, the adult is in complete control of the language learning situation. The adult controls the stimuli, how the child must respond, and all contingent behaviors based on the child's response. The second general approach is one in which the adults are trained to follow the child's lead and attend to items that interest the child. This is a more child-centered approach for parent training and is more consistent with the overall philosophy of intervention in this chapter. The child-centered approach reduces noncompliant behavior on the part of the child and enhances joint referencing between child and adult. These represent significant advantages in interaction styles.

McDade and Varnedoe (1987) suggest three component parts to parent training. First, the parents are trained to provide positive feedback to the child's communicative attempts. This involves teaching the parents to provide positive feedback in response to the child's verbalizations by acknowledging each communicative attempt. The parent is taught to demonstrate consistent recognition, praise, and recognition of the child's attempts to communicate (both verbal and nonverbal). The next aspect of parent training is teaching the parents how to use expansion as a facilitative technique. In this, parents are taught to expand all incomplete and grammatically incorrect utterances produced by the child. This technique facilitates grammatical development and increases the likelihood that the child will imitate the expanded utterance. The final suggestion relates to commenting strategies. Commenting strategies represent an intervention procedure, with the parents instructed to produce utterances (at the child's level) that provide new information. Commenting and expansion have proved to be effective intervention procedures and are an integral aspect of parent training.

The Hanen Approach

One of the most widely used and successful models for effectively training parents as language facilitators is the Hanen Early Language Parent Program (Girolometto, Greenburg, & Manolson, 1986). The Hanen Center, located in Toronto, Canada, has provided training to thousands of early interventionists throughout the world. The overall goal of the Hanen approach is to equip parents and primary caregivers to become better communicative partners. The approach is user friendly, relatively easy to learn, reflects the naturalistic manner in which language is learned, incorporates a conversational strategy, and promotes a child-centered model of intervention training. Additional information about the Hanen approach is provided by Manolson (1992), Manolson, Ward, and Dodington (1996), and Weitzman (1992).

An underlying tenet of the Hanen model is that the role of the adult is key to facilitating language learning in children. More specifically, an adult's responsiveness to a child's cues during all stages of communication development is paramount in encouraging greater communicative performance by the child. As the adult learns to follow the child's lead, the child is able to direct greater attention to the topic he or she chooses, rather than try to adapt to a topic chosen by the adult. For children with communication delay, dialogue skills are limited. Hence, the linguistic environment of the child is not able to optimally stimulate and enhance language development and performance. The Hanen program is a conversational model of language intervention that accepts and promotes dialogue skills as a prerequisite to communication development. Inherent in this model is the supposition that a child with well-developed dialogue skills is furnished increased opportunity to learn language.

The Hanen program consists of two modules. First, the focus is on assisting parents to identify the child's attempts to communicate. In addition, the parent is shown how to respond contingently. The second module involves training the parents to preplan play activities designed to encourage and enhance interactions between adult and child. Table 5–15 presents a summary of the Hanen program content (Girolometto et al., 1986).

TABLE 5–15   Outline of the Hanen Early Language Parent Program

Observe the Child's Attempts to Communicate

The objective is to increase parental awareness of a child's ability to communicate at all levels of communicative ability. Increased awareness of a child's attempts to communicate equips parents to adapt their responses to the child's communicative level.

Follow the Child's Lead

The objective is to increase the parents' responsiveness to their child's vocal, nonverbal, and verbal behaviors. Parents are exposed to strategies that enable them to respond to the child's communicative and potentially communicative initiations (topic initiations).

Respond So the Child Will Learn

The parents are taught to add information to the child's topic that is at the child's level. Response patterns the parents are exposed to include imitation, labeling, expansion, commenting, and clarification. Animation and repetition are encouraged.

Keep the Conversation Going—Take Turns

The overall objective is to improve the parents' ability to engage their children in joint activities for longer periods of time and thereby to take more turns on the same topic. Parents are taught signals that cue the child to stay in the conversation for more turns.

Prompt for Better Turns

Parents are taught how to provide their children with specific information needed to improve their turn-taking ability. The prompting must remain primarily within a child-centered framework.

Preplan Play Activities

Parents are taught how to preplan play activities that incorporate previously learned conversational strategies. Additional opportunities for dialogue are needed in addition to those available through the natural give-and-take of everyday interactions.

Adapted from "Developing Dialogue Skills: The Hanen Early Language Parent Program," by L. Girolometto, J. Greenburg, and A. Manolson, 1986, *Seminars in Speech and Language, 7*, p. 367.

Additional materials provided by the Hanen Center help parents identify a child's individual conversational style (Weitzman, 1992). Weitzman notes that typically developing children react differently to conversational opportunities. Hence, it is reasonable that children with delayed communication development will likewise reflect various conversational styles. It is important that interventionists and parents be aware of these styles and incorporate this knowledge into intervention activities. A summary of the conversational styles, as described by Weitzman, is presented in Table 5–16.

One final issue regarding the Hanen program deserves consideration at this point. Does it work? Is the approach adopted by the Hanen program effective in promoting parents/adults as language facilitators? The answer to that question appears to be yes. Girolometto et al. (1986) demonstrated that mothers who participated in the Hanen program adopted a conversational style that facilitated high levels of responsiveness, topic initiation, and turn taking in their children. Specifically, the mothers who participated were more con-

TABLE 5–16 Descriptions of Conversational Styles

The Sociable Child

The sociable child readily initiates interactions and shows increased responsiveness to adult interactions. This behavior may be noted in infancy. Even the child with communicative delay may show increased interest in interaction opportunities.

The Reluctant Child

This child seldom initiates and may choose to be on the outside of group activities. The child may require a warm-up period prior to responding to interaction attempts by peers or adults. The child with communication delay may show increased reluctance to interact due to a desire to avoid frustration at the lack of communicative ability.

The Child with His Own Agenda

This child shows little interest in interaction and may prefer to play alone. The child may initiate interactions when needing something but may frequently reject adult efforts to engage in turn taking. For the child with significant delay in communication development, this lack of interest in interaction may persist over time.

The Passive Child

This child seldom responds or initiates. Little interest in people or objects is noted. This child shows reluctance in participating in any type of interaction or turn-taking exchanges.

Adapted from *Learning Language and Loving It*, (p. 1), by E. Weitzman, 1992, Toronto, Canada: Hanen Center.

tingently responsive to their children's behavior and also reduced their topic control to a greater extent than the control group of mothers. As a result, their children were also more contingently responsive, initiated more topics, and ignored their mothers less often than the control group. In addition, they used more verbal turns and a more diverse vocabulary than the control group of children. The authors concluded that the program resulted in mothers' increased ability to follow the child's lead, and mothers provided increased contingent feedback; a more balanced turn-taking mode was noted, and longer conversational exchanges resulted. These results are significant and underscore the effectiveness of parent training activities.

Peer-Mediated Interventions

A powerful force in the development of age-appropriate communication skills is the effect of social relationships. Developing social relationships with one's peers is part of child development. For some children, particularly those with communication delay, acquiring the prerequisite social communication skills necessary for successful peer interactions is difficult. The EI may choose a child's peers as resources as part of communication-based intervention. Teaching typically developing children strategies to promote positive social-communication interactions with partners who display communication delay can be an important adjunct to communication-based intervention. Table 5–17 presents principles designed to guide the development of effective peer-mediated intervention (Ostrosky, Kaiser, & Odom, 1992). Formalized instruction provided for peers of communicatively delayed children is a relatively new intervention avenue. Although there is a moderate body of information supporting the efficacy of such an intervention strategy, more research is needed regarding the content of training and the general effectiveness of this approach.

CHAPTER SUMMARY

The process of communication development for typically developing children begins early, is predicated on environmental opportunity, involves communicative partners, and incorporates numerous aspects of a child's abilities to be complete. If the development process begins early, it is reasonable to assume that for those children displaying communication delay or those at risk of doing so, the process of intervention must likewise begin early. The entire early intervention team must be alert to the issues raised in this chapter if effective interven-

TABLE 5-17   Guidelines to Effective Peer-Mediated Intervention

• All types of peer interaction should be facilitated. This includes interaction between typically developing children and children with communication delay.

• All children must be taught social-communicative strategies to maximize the effects of intervention activities.

• Children should be chosen for peer-mediated instruction based, in part, on their potential for success.

• Children with delayed communication should initially receive individual instruction. The focus of this instruction should be conversational initiation and conversational response strategies.

• Instruction for typically developing children should revolve around conversational strategies that are known to elicit verbal and nonverbal behaviors from children with communication delay.

• A direct instruction approach should be used to teach desired social-communicative behaviors to all children.

• Maintenance and generalization must be consciously planned for in the intervention program adopted.

Adapted from "Facilitating Children's Social-Communicative Interactions through the Use of Peer-Mediated Interventions" (p. 310), by M. Ostrosky, A. Kaiser, and S. Odom in *Enhancing Children's Communication: Research Foundations for Intervention*, edited by A. Kaiser and D. Gray, 1992, Baltimore: Paul H. Brookes.

tion services are to be provided. Recall that the single best predictor of school success is communication skill. For the vast majority of children who are part of early intervention, the major area of disability they display is social-communicative development. It is imperative that parents and clinicians acknowledge the primacy of communication skills and direct full attention toward the prevention of problems as well as remediation for those children displaying communication disorders.

REFERENCES

Briggs, M. (1992, November). *Communication intervention for infants and toddlers: A family context approach*. Paper presented at the annual convention of the Wisconsin Speech-Language-Hearing Association, Oshkosh, WI.

Cartright, L., & Ruscello, D. (1979). A survey of parent involvement practices in the speech clinic. *ASHA, 21*, 275.

Devine, M. (1990). *Growing together: Communication activities for infants and toddlers*. Tucson, AZ: Communication Skill Builders.

Foster, S. (1985). The development of discourse topic skills by infants and young children. *Topics in Language Disorders, 5*, 31.

Girolometto, L., Greenburg, J., & Manolson, A. (1986). Developing dialogue skills: The Hanen early language parent program. *Seminars in Speech and Language, 4,* 367.

Keenan, E., & Schieffelin, B. (1976). Topic as a discourse notion: A study of topic in the conversation of children and adults. In C. Li (Ed.), *Subject and topic* (p. 90). New York: Academic Press.

Leonard, L. (1992). Communication intervention for young children at risk for specific communication disorders. *Seminars in Speech and Language, 13,* 223.

Linder, T. (1993). *Transdisciplinary play-based intervention.* Baltimore: Paul H. Brookes.

MacDonald, J., & Carroll, J. (1992). A partnership model for communicating with infants at risk. *Infants and Young Children, 4,* 20.

Manolson, A. (1992). *It takes two to talk.* Toronto, Canada: Hanen Center.

Manolson, A., Ward, B., & Dodington, N. (1996). *You make the difference.* Toronto, Canada: Hanen Center.

McDade, H., & Varnedoe, D. (1987). Training parents to be language facilitators. *Topics in Language Disorders, 7,* 19.

McLean, J., & Snyder-McLean, L. (1991). Application of pragmatics to severely mentally retarded children and youth. In R. Schiefelbusch & L. Lloyd (Eds.), *Language perspectives: Acquisition, retardation, and intervention* (p. 250). Austin, TX: PRO-ED.

Ostrosky, M., Kaiser, A., & Odom, S. (1992). Facilitating children's social-communicative interactions through the use of peer-mediated interventions. In A. Kaiser & D. Gray (Eds.), *Enhancing children's communication: Research foundations for intervention* (p. 100). Baltimore: Paul H. Brookes.

Patrick, S. (1993). Facilitating communication and language development. In T. Linder (Ed.), *Transdisciplinary play-based intervention* (p. 163). Baltimore: Paul H. Brookes.

Reidlich, C., & Herzfeld, M. (1983). *0–3 Years: An early language curriculum.* Moline, IL: LinguiSystems.

Spradlin, J., & Siegel, G. (1982). Language training in natural and clinical environments. *Journal of Speech and Hearing Disorders, 47,* 2.

Vellman, S., Davis, B., & Vihman, M. (1994, November). *Why do babies need speech therapy?* Paper presented at the annual convention of the American Speech-Language-Hearing Association, San Antonio, TX.

Weatherby, A., Cain, D., Yonclas, D., & Walker, V. (1988). Analysis of intentional communication of normal children from the prelinguistic to the multiword stage. *Journal of Speech and Hearing Research, 31,* 240.

Weatherby, A., & Prizant, B. (1989). The expression of communicative intent: Assessment guidelines. *Seminars in Speech and Language, 10,* 77.

Weitzman, E. (1992). *Learning language and loving it.* Toronto, Canada: Hanen Center.

Wilcox, J. (1989). Delivering communication-based services to infants, toddlers, and their families: Approaches and models. *Topics in Language Disorders, 10,* 68.

Yoder, P., & Warren, S. (1993). Can developmentally delayed children's language development be enhanced through prelinguistic intervention? In A. Kaiser & D. Gray (Eds.), *Enhancing children's communication: Research foundations for intervention* (p. 120). Baltimore: Paul H. Brookes.

APPENDIX 5–A COMMUNICATION
INTERVENTION MATERIALS

Beckman, P. (1996). *Strategies for working with families of young children with disabilities*. Baltimore: Paul H. Brookes.

Bricker, D. (1993). *Assessment, evaluation, and programming system for infants and children*. Baltimore: Paul H. Brookes.

Bricker, D. & Cripe, J. (1992). *An activity-based approach to early intervention*. Baltimore: Paul H. Brookes.

Cohen, L. (1996). *Child development, health, and safety*. Gaithersburg, MD: Aspen Publications.

Lampman, S. (1999). *Intervention strategies for infants and toddlers with special needs*. Columbus, OH: Prentice Hall.

Linder, T. (1993). *Transdisciplinary play-based intervention*. Baltimore: Paul H. Brookes.

MacDonald, J. (1997). *Before your child talks*. Tallmadge, OH: Family Child Learning Center.

MacDonald, J. (1997). *Communication partners collection*. Tallmadge, OH: Family Child Learning Center.

Manolson, A. (1992). *It takes two to talk*. Toronto, Canada: Hanen Center.

Manolson, A., Ward, B., & Dodington, N. (1996). *You make the difference*. Toronto, Canada: Hanen Center.

Parks, S. (Ed.). (1998). *Help at home*. Palo Alto, CA: Vort Corporation.

Santana, A., & Bottino, P. (1998). *Comprehensive early stimulation program for infants*. Detroit, MI: Wayne State University Press.

Supporting families of children with special needs. (1998). St. Louis, MO: Parents as Teachers National Center.

Weil, C. (1998). *Tips for teaching infants and toddlers*. Vero Beach, FL: The Speech Bin.

Weitzman, E. (1992). *Learning language and loving it*. Toronto, Canada: Hanen Center.

CHAPTER

6

Is Early Intervention Effective?

ℭℭ *Clinicians, administrators, legislators, physicians, local school district personnel, researchers, and parents have invested a significant amount of time, effort, and resources into establishing a comprehensive program of early intervention services for at-risk children, children with disabilities, and their families. The stakes are high. The potential benefit of effective services is great, and the impact on families is substantial. All these resources are directed toward positively impacting the lives of children. All concerned professionals are interested in answering one very important question:* **Is early intervention effective?** **"**

In 1974 Urie Bronfenbrenner raised a significant question regarding the efficacy of early intervention. He asked, in a now-famous monograph, "Is early intervention effective?" It has been 26 years since that question was posed. Researchers from all academic disciplines are still demonstrating the efficacy of the services provided to at-risk and disabled children and their families. Much has changed in the early intervention enterprise since then. More effective models of service delivery, new legislative mandates, emerging disciplines, better training, new curricula, fresh certification and accreditation standards, increased funding, better assessment techniques, and enhanced medical technology have changed the landscape of early intervention. And yet, the question remains, "Is early intervention effective?"

In the present climate of aggressive family-focused intervention for infants and toddlers who are at risk, perhaps the efficacy question should be altered. The past 25 years of research on the effectiveness of early intervention has resulted in a relatively clear answer to the efficacy question: **Yes, early intervention is effective.** However, the question regarding efficacy must be rephrased. Perhaps the question, "Does early intervention work?" should be changed to, "For whom does it work and under what circumstances?" Greater specificity in the efficacy question will increase our knowledge of how to intervene with young children and their families. As federal, state, and local funding for early intervention services expands over the years, questions about the effectiveness of services will be raised with increasing frequency.

Historically, efficacy has been measured in the context of child change. Child change is the amount of (measurable) developmental progress or change a child demonstrates over time as a result of intervention services. Child change is determined by comparing developmental assessment results at two points in time. Generally, the child is assessed at the outset of intervention. Following a period of intervention, the child is reassessed. The difference between the initial assessment and the final assessment has historically been attributed to the intervention provided. Thus, when positive results are noted, the early interventionist expresses pleasure with the efficacy of services. One possible response to change noted over time might be, "Thank goodness for maturation!" In other words, past research on efficacy has not consistently demonstrated the effectiveness of intervention apart from the effects of maturation, and for some children child change may not be the best measure of efficacy. Recall that age, time, and maturation are on the child's side. Thus, children tend to change, even without intervention. A more careful look at child change over time, apart from maturation, must be undertaken if the efficacy question is to be fully answered.

The material in this chapter is designed to provide information to assist in answering the efficacy question. A broad array of research findings will be discussed. The tables are devised to provide all EI personnel with a ready reference of data regarding efficacy, regardless of setting, populations served, service delivery model, developmental domains measured, or professionals involved. It is anticipated that the information in this chapter will better equip the EI to answer the continuing and important question, "Is early intervention working?"

BEST PRACTICE

"Best practice" is one concept relating to efficacy that all EIs should become familiar with. The concept of best practice is not new. In fact,

references to best practice can be seen in the special education literature since the early 1980s (Peters & Heron, 1992). Although use of the
term best practice is widespread, a clear definition of the term is hard
to come by. Initially, the concept was used in the context of services to
people who were severely impaired. As such, definitions of best practice included references to age-appropriate skills, independent living,
methods used to deliver educational services, and quality of life. Over
a relatively short period of time, the concept of best practice shifted
from the usage of age-appropriate skills across settings, to strategies
and methods, delivery of instruction, and quality of life outcomes. The
concept of best practice shifted from student (skills needed) to the
instruction (method) and back to the student (outcomes produced).

Best practice in the context of early intervention is harder to identify. The primary focus of efficacy has shifted from child-centered measures to a family focus, making efficacy more elusive to document and
demonstrate. Meyer and Eichinger (1987) have suggested that the concept of "most promising practices" be considered. Most promising
practices are referred to as exemplary and innovative developments,
generated by applied research efforts and designed to validate effective
strategies of intervention. The concept of most promising suggests that
identified practices are potentially powerful but may require ongoing
empirical investigation for support. Additional terms such as "emerging strategies" and "exemplary strategies" can be found in the early
intervention literature, as well. In essence, these terms and concepts are
functionally equivalent to best practice. Best practice represents an
effort to integrate and synthesize emerging empirical data into everyday application. As such, this practice will never cease. Searching for
best practice draws attention to the multiple variables that must be considered and studied, experimented with, and integrated into early
intervention services. The result will be qualitative changes in the lives
of children and their families. The discussion that follows is designed
to alert the EI to an array of issues that facilitate best practice, thus
resulting in an overall increase in the efficacy of services provided.

GENERAL EFFICACY CONSIDERATIONS

The provision of timely and efficacious early intervention services for
infants and toddlers who are at risk or displaying special needs and
their families is of paramount concern to a growing array of professionals. One common frustration, voiced by many EI personnel, is that
early access to children is denied them. Perhaps one of the reasons
why early access is denied is because of their inability to answer the

efficacy question. Of all the areas in which the EI must become a broker of information, perhaps none is more important than issues surrounding the effectiveness of services.

Any discussion of efficacy can be subdivided into several branches. However, a careful review of existing literature seems to divide efficacy literature into two distinct categories, with subheadings under each. That is to say, the existing literature suggests that the efficacy of services provided to children under 3 years, particularly if child-change measures are employed to measure effectiveness, is dependent on two primary factors. These are age of identification and caregiver involvement. That is to say, those children identified early and those children whose caregivers are involved in the provision of intervention demonstrate a better overall outcome. Children with established disabilities who receive early intervention services early (under 3 years) have overall better outcomes than those children for whom intervention is delayed (Shonkoff & Hauser-Cram, 1987). In addition, the provision of services as early as possible can be preventive. Secondary complications, inherent in later identification and relating to both the child and the family, can be minimized with early intervention.

What this means to the EI is that anything that can be done to improve age of identification and anything that might be done to increase the likelihood that parents will be involved in early intervention will generally result in a better level of development for the child. Earlier chapters (Chapters 1 and 2) provided ample information to help the EI maximize the potential for earlier identification as well as optimize the involvement of significant adults.

Guralnick and Bennett (1987), based on 25 years of experience in research, program development, and service provision, suggest that the value of providing early intervention for children and families is well established. Parents and service providers continue to testify to the effect of early intervention on children and families. Several broad and more specific statements may be made about child change and family change.

Child Change

The range of effects and benefits of early intervention is impressive. Positive outcomes have been documented for children born at biological risk (premature, low-birth-weight children); children from families stressed by the absence of social supports, personal problems, or limited financial resources; and children with established developmental disabilities (Casto & Mastropieri, 1986; Farran, 1990; Guralnick, 1988, 1997; Guralnick & Bennett, 1987; Ramey & Ramey, 1992; Shonkoff & Hauser-Cram, 1987).

It has been well documented that comprehensive early intervention programs (multifaceted and integrated child development with family focus) can be effective in reducing the overall decline in developmental status that is observed in the first few years of life for children at biological risk and for those from severely disadvantaged families (Bennett & Guralnick, 1992; Bryant & Ramey, 1987; Infant Health and Development Program, 1990). Positive effects of early intervention have been obtained for children with established developmental disabilities, including those with communication disorders, visual impairments, hearing loss, motor deficits, and general cognitive delay (Guralnick & Bricker, 1987; Harris, 1987; Meadow-Orlans, 1987; Olson, 1987; Snyder-McLean & McLean, 1987).

Different disciplines define the success of the services they provide in different ways. Thus, it is quite difficult to identify a universally accepted criterion that can be used to gauge the effectiveness of services, particularly when multiple professionals are providing services for the child. Table 6–1 provides an overview of how varying

TABLE 6–1   Evaluation/Efficacy Emphasis for Varying Disciplines

Profession	Emphasis	Criteria
Medicine	Physical health	Height and weight gain, absence of disease
Psychology	Age-appropriate development	Standardized assessment of developmental milestones
Physical and occupational therapy	Motor function	Clinical assessment of reflex control, quality of movement in mobility and self-care
Speech therapy	Communication	Assessment of functional speech and language skills
Social work	Social environment	Family functioning/ relationships
Mental health	Coping and daily function	Ability to handle stress and life in general
Teachers	Educational progress	Attainment of teaching goals
Administrators	Program planning	Meets educational mandates as required by state/federal law

Adapted from *Implementing Early Intervention*, by C. Tingey, 1989, Baltimore: Paul Brookes.

disciplines might define efficacy. As will be noted, measurable criteria are difficult to agree upon because skills cross disciplinary boundaries and expertise.

The Infant Health and Development Project (1990) cited previously demonstrated that child change, as measured by standard scores on child development measures, was greater for children receiving home-based early intervention up to 12 months of age followed by center-based early intervention services up to age 3 years. In addition, a family-based intervention program in the United States and an additional program in Sweden have likewise demonstrated significant benefits of early intervention services for children under the age of 3 years (Meyer, Coll, & Lester, 1994; Westrup, Klebeg, & Hugo, 1999). Lee & Kahn (1997) further demonstrated the efficacy of such services and state that "with the public and political outcry for accountability, we must be able to demonstrate the effectiveness of early intervention." This data suggests quite clearly that early intervention effects positive child change. The "best practice" of service delivery appears to be home-based services up to 1 year of age and a combination of home- and center-based services from 1 year to 3 years. Further, home-based services are most efficacious when initiated early, provided on a regular basis (minimum of twice per month), and delivered in a transdisciplinary manner.

Family Change

Families have also benefited from early intervention programs, although this facet of efficacy is much more difficult to assess, particularly in light of the changing nature of families. It is well established that the responsibilities and demands of having a young child with developmental problems contribute to parental stress. Recent research has demonstrated that the adverse effects on family functioning can be minimized through family-focused, community-based support and services (Innocenti, Huh, & Boyce, 1992; Mahoney, O'Sullivan, & Robinson, 1992; Orr, Cameron, Dobson, & Day, 1993). These studies consistently demonstrate that several variables related to family functioning remain essentially unchanged in the presence of a young child with disability, providing that family support systems are in place. Other aspects of family adjustment, including depression, sense of competence, relationship with one's spouse, feelings of attachment to the child, degree of social isolation, and parental health are minimally affected if appropriate family intervention is provided. As mentioned in earlier chapters, the EI can no longer afford to view the child as the "client." In a very real sense, the entire family is receiving services of one type or another. Although these services are harder to measure and quantify, for many families they are the most beneficial aspect of early intervention. Families readily acknowledge that in some instances (due to the nature of the child's problems), minimal change will be seen in the child. However, these same families frequently report that the intervention the family received was a lifesaver for them. This point cannot be understated. For many families, the EI is the lifeline to the outside world and provides ongoing encouragement and support.

Recent research involving children at risk and those with established disabilities supports the shift toward family-centered services. For example, the adverse developmental outcomes associated with prematurity are lessened to a substantial degree through early intervention programs that have focused on enhancing the quality of parent-child interactions as well as parents' feelings of competence and confidence (Guralnick, 1989; Resnick, Armstrong, & Carter, 1988). Additional efficacy studies have suggested that parents' self-perceptions of competence and confidence are fostered over time by family-focused early intervention. This helps parents cope with the obvious and more subtle problems that arise during stress periods in a child's development. Early intervention has the potential to strengthen the families' ability to undergo necessary adjustments (Achenbach, Howell, Aoki, & Rauh, 1993; Achenbach, Phares, Howell, Rauh, & Nurcombe, 1990). Shonkoff and Hauser-Cram (1987) have suggested that early intervention activities that concurrently involve both the child and the family are superior to those directed separately to participants. Parent-child relationships are integral to developmental progress on the child's part. Thus, efforts to help the parents understand the child's intentional communication cues and attempts to enhance reciprocal and contingent parent-child interaction are important (Seifer, Clark, & Sameroff, 1991). McCollum (1991) likewise suggests that activities of this nature do make a difference. Put simply, the child must receive all early intervention services in the context of the family. Both the child and family benefit if services are provided with this in mind.

Early intervention has also been effective when social supports are provided for families. Support provided by relatives, friends, parent groups, the clergy, and other professionals is generally associated with enhanced family functioning. Family-driven services (matching family needs with intervention) also strengthen collaborative relationships within the family (Patterson & McCubbin, 1983). Providing family support during stressful periods can increase attachment between parents and their children. This is important because lack of proper attachment has long-term implications for children's cognitive and social development (Belsky, 1984) and likely increases the potential that the family will continue as important contributors to the child's intervention activities. In families with young children who are disabled, early attachment formation can readily be compromised. Chapter 2 provided a variety of suggestions for the EI interested in minimizing the potential for attachment difficulties for parents of young children with special needs.

EFFICACY IN THE NEONATAL INTENSIVE CARE NURSERY

Ongoing advances in neonatology have allowed for the survival of increasing numbers of infants who would not have survived even 5 years ago. It is precisely because of these advances in the medical care of premature newborns that attention is shifting more toward improving the developmental outcome of these survivors. In other words, infants are surviving today who would have never survived previously, and we are now equally concerned with their quality of life following hospital discharge.

Previously presented information suggested that the earlier intervention begins, the better. It is hard to identify a setting earlier than the intensive care nursery (NICU) in which to initiate family-centered services. For those interested in the efficacy of NICU-based services, it must be recalled that there are three basic avenues of service provision. Intervention activities may be directed toward the infant, toward the family, or toward the staff. There is emerging literature regarding the effectiveness of intervention provided in each of these three areas. The available literature identifies both short- and long-term benefits of intervention that begins in the nursery. In addition, there is evidence of the benefit of such services for both the infant and the family. Table 6–2 summarizes various studies that address NICU-based intervention.

What these and other investigations reveal is that NICU-based intervention has a positive effect both for the infants and the caregivers. Attention directed toward caregivers primarily provides them with sufficient information so that the nursery is less aversive to them. Chapter 2 indicated that parents frequently report that the atmosphere of the NICU resulted in their adopting a posture of helplessness and that they felt "out of the loop" in the exchange of information among the NICU staff. As a result of these reports, NICU policies have changed markedly in the past 10 to 15 years. Parents are now afforded

TABLE 6-2 Efficacy of NICU-Based Intervention

Reference	Intervention	Children Studied	Outcome
Katz, 1971	Auditory stimulation	62 infants; 28–32 weeks GA	E group higher in general maturation
Segall, 1972	Auditory stimulation	60 infants; 28–32 weeks GA	E group higher heart rate (more alert)
Powell, 1974	Tactile stimulation	36 infants between 1,000 and 2,000 g	Faster weight gain; higher BSID scores
Korner et al., 1975	Tactile stimulation	21 infants < 34 weeks GA	E group less apnea
Barnard, 1973	Tactile stimulation	15 infants; 28–32 weeks GA	E group greater gain in quiet sleep; greater neurologic maturation
Burns et al., 1983	Tactile stimulation	22 infants; 28–32 weeks GA	E group better motoric organization
Kramer & Pierpont, 1976	Tactile stimulation	20 infants < 34 weeks GA	E group better weight gain; increased head size
Rice, 1977	Tactile/vestibular	29 infants < 37 weeks GA	E group higher on Bayley mental scale
Rosenfield, 1980	Tactile	70 infants < 1,500 g	E group increased state organization; higher maternal visitation
White & Labarba, 1976	Tactile/kinesthetic	12 infants < 36 weeks GA	E group greater weight
Leib et al., 1980	Visual/tactile/ vestibular/auditory	28 infants between 1,200 and 1,800 g	E group higher on Bayley motor and mental scales
Grunwald & Becker, 1991	Staff education/ parent training	Staff and parents of infants in NICU	E group better respiratory status; better feeding; better behavioral organization

(continued)

TABLE 6-2 (continued)

Reference	Intervention	Children Studied	Outcome
Resnick et al., 1987	Tactile/vestibular/ kinesthetic/auditory/ visual/parent education	*255 infants, 500–1,800 g	E group higher mental and physical development
Becker et al., 1991	Staff education	21 infants < 1,500 g	E group better feeding; enhanced respiration; shorter hospitalization; improved behavioral organization; positive changes in nursing routine
Blanchard, 1991**	Various intervention modalities	Various populations	E group's reduction of stress better medical outcome; shorter stay in hospital and on respirator; better feeding; better weight gain; lower % of IVH; higher developmental scores
Wilson et al., 1994	Staff training	NICU staff	Improved level of developmentally appropriate care
Als et al., 1994	Individualized developmental care	LBW premature infants	E group shorter time on respirator; reduced BPD; reduced IVH; better developmental outcome
Heriza & Sweeney, 1990**	Various intervention modalities	Various populations	E group's developmental improvement; better developmental scores; better behavioral organization; reduced startle; increased quiet sleep

Achenbach et al., 1993*	Parent training	24 LBW children	E group had better long-term developmental outcome
Parker et al., 1991	Parent training	Infants < 36 weeks GA	E group had improved Bayley mental/motor scores
Jacobsen et al., 1988	Parent training	Mothers of LBW infants	E group showed increased interaction with infants at discharge and 4 weeks post-discharge

* Supplemented by home-based intervention

** Literature review study

BPD	Bronchopulmonary dysplasia
BSID	Bayley Scale of Infant Development
E group	Experimental group
GA	Gestational age
IVH	Intraventricular hemorrhage
LBW	Low birth weight

more autonomy than ever before. Several investigators have reported that parents, following greater involvement in the NICU, are more likely to participate in developmental follow-up programs, including programs of home visiting. These results appear to be most powerful among populations of mothers of low socioeconomic status. In such instances the benefit is twofold. The infant shows increased developmental performance and the family is more likely to be part of comprehensive intervention services following discharge.

Another recent development in providing NICU-based intervention has been "kangaroo care." This procedure is receiving increased acceptance in NICUs around the world. It gives the mother (fathers may also participate) and the infant an opportunity to experience more intense and direct skin-to-skin contact. Although there are variations in the amount of swaddling time and the specific methods employed, the procedure is essentially the same across hospitals: the mother strips to the waist and the infant is placed on her chest, with the two swaddled together. Although a substantial database on efficacy is emerging, early information suggests greater weight gain on the part of the child, with some reports suggesting an earlier release from the hospital. Further, mothers report positively on such programs. These reports indicate that the mother is less likely to struggle with her adequacy as a caregiver once the child transitions into the home setting.

Instruction provided to the NICU staff has also proven beneficial, both to mothers and infants. It must be recalled that the nature of the nursery itself mediates against the implementation of developmentally appropriate care. The nursery is not a nice place to begin the process of making sense of the world. However, changes in lighting, noise level, type and amount of touch, amount of interaction between adults and infants, and general procedures have affected both child and caregiver. Barba and Walker (1992) provide a framework for implementing a staff program with a more developmentally appropriate posture toward NICU care. It should be recalled that the NICU is a difficult environment in which to work. Staff turnover is higher than in many other nursing settings. Hence, the EI interested in providing developmentally appropriate care in the NICU is presented with an ongoing opportunity to forge relationships with the staff, provide important information, and implement changes in developmental practices as new procedures emerge. In other words, the need for training the staff never ceases. It is imperative that the hospital-based EI keep abreast of advances in the setting and scope of the NICU. NICU-based developmental specialists are increasing in number, with their scope of activity increasing also. Many developmental specialists desire access to the

NICU. Many more, currently working in the NICU, wonder about their role and scope of activity.

Perhaps an example from the author's experience can best demonstrate the posture that should be adopted in implementing developmentally appropriate procedures in a NICU, particularly a NICU that has been reluctant, for whatever reason, to move in the direction promoted.

Following a move into a new community, I was concerned that I would not be afforded the degree of access to infants and parents in the NICU that I had enjoyed in another state. I immediately applied for hospital staff privileges and began the process of gaining access to the NICU. No previous developmental specialists had been involved in NICU services. Soon after arriving in the new community, I met the chief of neonatal medicine. He was interested in implementing developmentally appropriate procedures in the NICU but was uncertain about how to proceed. He invited me into the nursery to provide a brief in-service for the nursing staff. The in-service lasted barely 30 minutes and contained very basic information on issues to consider as a move toward developmentally appropriate care was being considered. I spent the bulk of the day observing the NICU and becoming acquainted with procedures. Following the brief in-service and while leaving the NICU, I overheard two nurses talking. They were discussing the content of the in-service and were unaware that I was able to hear them, as I was hidden behind a coatrack. Nurse A said to Nurse B, "He seems like a very nice man, but I hope he does not expect us to change too much too soon."

The lesson is obvious. Early interventionists, although strongly encouraged to become brokers of information, are likewise encouraged to monitor how information is shared and how quickly changes are expected. The efficacy of NICU-based early intervention is well established. Specific changes in caregiving routine, the environment of the NICU, and parental participation in caregiving are possible. However, the manner in which changes are suggested, the timing of recommended changes, and the nature of the relationship between the EI and decision makers in the NICU may make or break the EI's ability to implement desired changes.

Services delivered to parents are varied and are an important facet of NICU-based care. Parents tell us that they desire information and assistance in attaching to their child. They also tell us they desire general support in adapting to the child they have, as opposed to the child they thought they might have. Although all mothers report some degree of apprehension about what might go wrong during their pregnancy, few indicate that this fear was maintained throughout their pregnancy. Thus, the child they feared has now become their reality. Mothers indicate consistently that they need help with this process. This is a difficult process for fathers as well. Although perhaps more reluctant to discuss these issues initially, fathers need assistance in adapting their expectations to the presence of a child with established or increased risk for developmental delay. The NICU-based EI is in a unique position to help parents adapt to these realities. Although harder to measure, the efficacy of parent-directed NICU intervention is substantial and has a long-lasting impact upon the child, parents, and overall family functioning. In the author's experience, this may be the best and most important role the EI plays. I continue to receive numerous letters and cards, some 2 to 4 years after the child was dismissed from the NICU, expressing deep appreciation for the manner in which the parents were assisted through their NICU experience.

Perhaps the most direct support of NICU-based intervention has been provided by VandenBerg (1996). In an important study that reviewed currently available research on the efficacy of NICU-based intervention, VandenBerg made the following points:

- Researchers have shifted their attention from improving survival rates for high-risk infants in NICUs to studying ways to improve developmental outcome.
- Available studies reviewing the efficacy of developmentally appropriate care in the NICU have demonstrated not only improved developmental outcome but also dramatically improved medical benefits and impressive cost savings.
- It is time that nurseries develop this type of care (developmentally appropriate care) for premature infants. NICUs choosing not to implement this type of therapy should have clear reasons and should consider their own randomized trials to attempt to disprove this work.
- **Developmental care is no longer optional. It is mandatory if we are to provide optimal care for low-birth-weight infants and those surviving the NICU.**

EFFICACY OF HOME-BASED INTERVENTION

The Transition Home

One of the primary distinctions of the legislation under which early intervention services are provided is mandated family involvement in the process. An important by-product of this has been the growing realization that family involvement and child change may be best facilitated if initial intervention services are provided in the home setting.

Transitions can be quite difficult for many families. This is particularly true when it comes time for the child to move from the hospital to the home setting. EI providers should be particularly sensitive to this transition, particularly if home-based services are to be initiated. When children are dismissed from the NICU or the pediatric intensive care unit, families must adapt their home environment and scheduling to meet the health and developmental needs of the child. Once medical transitions are completed, the family must then adapt to the specific and varied developmental needs presented by the child. Efficacy is significantly enhanced if careful hospital discharge planning is completed prior to the child going home. As stated previously, home-based services must begin early after discharge, be provided consistently (at least 2 times per month), involve the caregiver, and involve varied professionals functioning in a transdisciplinary mode.

Chapter 3 provided several reasons why the home setting is helpful for assessment. These same principles apply to home-based intervention. What has emerged over the past 10 years appears to be an early intervention service delivery system characterized by initial home visiting, followed by combined home and center services, which are followed by primarily center-based intervention provided by the public schools or other agencies. The home-visiting models currently employed allow for visits to begin early, preferably shortly after hospital discharge. In addition, home-visiting services are characterized by a transdisciplinary model of intervention. That is to say, there is one primary interventionist. The efficacy literature does not support the involvement of one discipline over another, particularly before the child reaches 1 year of age. The home visitor may represent one of any of the disciplines involved in early intervention. The available curricula stress a twofold approach to home-based intervention. The targets of intervention services are the child and the family. In essence, the home visitor provides instruction to the caregivers relative to the unique characteristics of their child with special needs and provides direct intervention for the child. In general, evaluation of early intervention programs that use home visiting demonstrates that these programs can improve both the short- and long-term health and well-being of families and children. Compared to families without access to home visiting, home-visited children display more age-appropriate developmental performance.

The following discussion provides specific information about the effectiveness of home visiting; the statements summarize several important investigations regarding home visiting.

- Children at risk of developmental delay have benefited from services delivered through home visiting. Premature, low-birth-weight babies and malnourished children whose families were seen by home visitors were able to physically and developmentally demonstrate "catch-up growth" (Field, 1980; Rauh, 1988; Ross, 1984).
- Fewer low-birth-weight children in a home-visiting program needed additional services after completing a 2-year program of home visiting when compared to children who had received no services (Resnick, Eyler, Nelson, Eitzman, & Bucciarelli, 1987).
- Three years following a home-visiting program, children in Jamaica demonstrated higher IQ scores than matched children who had received no home-based intervention (Grantham-McGregor, 1987).
- The cognitive development of rural and inner-city children who have received home-based early intervention is significantly above that of children who do not receive such services (Bryant & Ramey, 1987).
- Evaluations of early intervention programs using home visiting and varying in service intensity (the amount of program contact with clients over time) found that more intense programs are generally more effective.
- Intensive home visiting, in conjunction with medical and educational interventions, has proven effective at keeping developmental scores of groups of randomly assigned, disadvantaged children from dropping over time, compared to scores of controls. A comparative evaluation of 17 programs, 11 of which used home visiting, showed that program effectiveness increased as other services were combined with home visiting. Two of the three most effective and most intensive programs used home visiting in addition to center-based services (Bryant & Ramey, 1987).
- Home visiting appears to be more effective if begun early after discharge from the hospital and if characterized by one primary visitor making frequent visits (Heincke, Beckwith, & Thompson, 1989).
- Home visiting has resulted in increased social conversational skills in children who are developmentally delayed (Girolometto, 1988).
- Home visiting results in long-term benefits in overall developmental progress for children who are biologically at risk, when compared to children who do not receive home-based

intervention. Language skills and perceptual-motor skills are more likely to be delayed in children who are not involved in early home intervention (Berrera, Kitching, Cunningham, Douchet, & Rosenbaum, 1990).

● One review of the efficacy of home-based intervention has revealed that developmental intervention for infants at biological risk following hospital discharge can have positive effects. In general, the effectiveness of early home-based intervention is best demonstrated by differences in the home environment; increased responsivity and sensitivity by mothers on interaction measures; and, to a lesser degree, increased scores on cognitive measures (Sandall, 1990).

● Support provided to mothers by home visitors resulted in their displaying more favorable patterns of mother-infant interaction. The effect is most pronounced among teen and Hispanic women in low socioeconomic groups (Dawson et al., 1990).

In a national survey of nearly 2,000 home-visiting programs (Roberts & Wasik, 1989), 34% reported serving children under 3 years of age. The primary reason why these programs served children under 3 years was that the children were at risk for developmental delay or had already displayed delayed patterns of development of differing origin. These programs suggested that the primary rationale of home visits was to provide support to parents or to teach parenting skills, with reduction in parental stress as a secondary reason. Many of these programs reported that they incorporate the modeling of positive adult-child interactions, provide direct child-centered intervention, and include appropriate learning activities in the home-based curricula.

Home visiting is a flexible, cost-effective strategy for observing and teaching families about the special needs of their children. The need for support, particularly from a professional familiar with the issues faced by parents of children with special needs, may be best met through home visiting. The home-visit model has the potential to serve families and children with established conditions, as well as those at increased risk of developing delayed patterns of development. Home visiting has proven to be an effective method of positively impacting the lives of children with special needs and their families.

EFFICACY OF HOME-CENTER PROGRAMS

The emerging model for effective early intervention services for children under 3 years of age appears to be a combination of home-based and center-based services. The following information provides efficacy data for combination home-center intervention. Combination home-center programs provide initial intervention in the home for a specified period. Once the home-based facet of the program is completed (usually determined by the child's chronological age, generally between 12 and 18 months of age), the center-based component is added. For the most part, home-based services are provided until the child reaches 1 year of age. Many programs go slightly longer. Programs that provide primarily home-based services longer than 1 year tend to be in geographic regions in which center-based services are not readily available. There has been a more recent trend to provide home-based services exclusively until the child reaches age 3. This trend is not supported in the efficacy literature. There are significant advantages to center-based services for the child past 1 year of age. These advantages extend to both the child and the family.

The discussion that follows primarily covers the center-based component of early intervention services. Center-based service systems, regardless of whether a home-based component is included or not, tend to cluster into several distinct categories. These include parent-child centers, specialized (developmental) child-care centers, and medical child-care centers.

In parent-child centers, mothers spend varying amounts of time in the center with their children. The mothers attend meetings, participate in child development classes, and receive direct instruction on how they might better facilitate their child's development as well as cope with the stresses inherent in having a child with special needs. Parent-child programs most likely provide group intervention for the children. The staff leads the group in activities designed to promote the children's development and provide support for the mothers.

Developmental child-care intervention settings serve children birth through school age. Centers of this nature are found across the United States. In these settings, the primary focus of intervention is the child. Services are provided in the center and away from the child's home. Primary emphasis is not directed toward parent training, although some attention is given to parents. In an idealized form, developmental child care for children with special needs involves intervention provided by competent, trained staff in classes with low staff-child ratios, which are housed in a developmentally appropriate environment. Children with a high level of developmental need may best be served through this model, perhaps following a home-based component. This model can offer intervention services of a relatively high intensity.

One final model of center-based intervention is the medical child-care model. For some children with pressing medical and developmental needs, a medical child-care/developmental intervention model is best. In settings of this nature, a child spends the bulk of his or her time in a specialized setting with appropriate staff expertise to meet the serious medical needs the child might have. These programs can serve families with a wide variety of needs: family support, medical support, respite care, parent support groups, and educational opportunities. These services are all provided in concert with an individualized intervention program for each child. In the context of the styles of center-based intervention just described, Table 6–3 identifies a variety of investigations specifying populations studied and the outcomes obtained. What emerges is a clear and concise picture that strengthens support for the effectiveness of early intervention. Services provided for children under 3 years of age that are begun early, include parental involvement, have a home- and center-based component, and allow for the highest quality of intervention activities do make a difference in the lives of children and families. This effect is seen across socioeconomic strata, cultural groups, and developmental domains.

COST EFFICACY

Providing effective early intervention services comes with a price, not the least of which is financial. Some argue that the most obvious and readily measured economic aspect of early intervention is program cost, not only the cost of implementing early intervention programs but cost savings over time as a result of doing so. In other words, does early intervention save money over what later remediation educational costs might be? How much a program costs and cost savings over time are critical considerations for decision makers at all levels.

Barnett (1993) has provided some helpful information in analyzing the cost benefits resulting from preschool intervention programs. Although the Barnett data centered primarily on children growing up in poverty, many of the results are applicable to the populations of children discussed in this text. General findings in the Barnett investigation indicate that the study's preschool education program produced economic benefits to participants and to the general public. Further, these benefits greatly exceed the overall costs of the preschool program. The Barnett data suggests a 7:1 ratio between dollars expended and long-term benefit to participants and society in general. He suggests that not many federally funded programs could generate ratios so favorable. The 7:1 cost-benefit ratio described by Barnett is not significantly out of line with other figures reported in the literature. Home Visiting (1990) points out that one preschool program estimated that every dollar spent on preschool intervention saves from $3

TABLE 6-3 Efficacy of Primarily Center-Based Intervention

Reference	Children Studied	Outcome
Girolometto et al., 1986	20 preschool DD children	Improved maternal responsiveness to child's cues; improved child language skills
MacDonald & Carroll, 1992	Preschool language delayed	Improved overall communication skills
Fewell & Delwein, 1991	Mentally retarded; other DD	E groups showed significant gains over control group
Bruder, 1993	30 DD children	Significant gains for all children
Macfarland-Smith et al., 1993	DD toddlers	Significant gains in object ID
Johnson & Walker, 1991	1- to 3-year-old Hispanic	Significant gains in school readiness
Martin et al., 1990	Infants at risk of DD	IQ scores higher than controls
Solomon, 1995*	Various populations	Socially disadvantaged children helped; family adaptation and functioning improved; increased child potential; effective programs begin early; comprehensive programs more effective; highly structured programs more effective; children who receive EI services require less special education; EI works for children and families
Ramey & Ramey, 1992	LBW premature infants	Positive outcomes for E group
Spiker et al., 1993	LBW premature, at risk	Improved maternal-child interaction
Brookes-Gunn et al., 1992	LBW infants	E group had higher cognitive scores at 24 and 36 months

TABLE 6–3 *(continued)*

Reference	Children Studied	Outcome
Fey & Cleave, 1990	Language-delayed children	E groups have higher language scores than control groups
Pinder & Olswang, 1995	CP children	E group higher communication skills
IHDP, 1990	LBW children	E group higher overall developmental scores
Markowitz et al., 1991	489 children in EI before age 5 years	E group scored higher in all areas; gains were greater than maturation

*: Review study
CP: Cerebral palsy
DD: Developmentally delayed
E group: Experimental group
IHDP: Infant Health and Development Program
LBW: Low birth weight

to $6 later on. This represents a cost savings ratio from 3:1 to 6:1. An additional study reported in Home Visiting (1990) suggested that, on average, $1,100 less was spent on school remedial services for boys who received preschool intervention services. Roberts (1991) likewise reports that early intervention programs save money. The Committee for Economic Development (1987) listed the cost-benefit ratio for early intervention programs to be 4:1. Miller (1987) also lists cost benefits resulting from early intervention activities. Rossetti (1990) provides additional data regarding the cost effectiveness of early intervention programs. It is widely acknowledged that costs of special education exceed those of regular education. In 1984, the average annual cost per child for regular education in the United States ranged from $1,148 to $2,060 per child. Thus, the average cost per child for regular education to age 18 ranged from $13,776 to $16,072. In contrast, the average cost for special education to age 18, when intervention starts at birth, age 2, and age 6, is $32,273, $37,600, and $48,816, respectively. Further, the median cost of special education per child per year in 1981 was reported to be $2,012 for infants, $2,310 for preschoolers, and $4,445 for elementary and secondary students (Rossetti, 1990a). More recently, Rossetti (1990a) reported that special education costs rose 10% between 1977 and 1985, with regular education costs rising only 4% during the same period. Variations in cost benefits are caused by many factors, including the type of services provided, the setting in which services are delivered, the amount of services, and the number of staff involved. Regardless of these variables, early intervention saves money in the long term. In addition, families that participate in early intervention realize economic benefits that are indirectly attributable to intervention. Enhanced school performance affords children improved job potential and, hence, increased earnings potential.

The discussion supporting early intervention becomes more favorable when economic benefits are considered. At the least, measurable savings can be realized if parents are better able to meet the needs of their child at home, thus avoiding the need for institutional or more involved (expensive) care. There are considerable savings in educational costs because early intervention increases the likelihood of regular education placement. A savings also is realized for children who need long-term special education services if intervention begins early. In addition, parents of children with special needs are enabled to become more self-sufficient. On the whole, economic benefits accrue as a result of services provided for young children who are at risk and disabled.

THE CHALLENGE TO EARLY INTERVENTIONISTS

In a climate of increasing fiscal accountability to the public and funding agencies, all EI personnel must be concerned with efficacy. It is not enough anymore to simply say that EI activities work. Documentation, data, comparative information, empirical comparisons, and hard facts must be provided to policy makers. This data is best provided by those most directly involved in early intervention activities. After all, "hands-on" clinicians, those who see firsthand the benefit to families and children and are eyewitnesses to the power of early intervention, are in the best position to address the efficacy question. In many instances, EI professionals become so involved in "sharpening our clinical skills" that they overlook the need to demonstrate the effectiveness of services. This must not be allowed to continue. It is not simply the domain of the researcher to demonstrate efficacy. It is the responsibility of all intervention providers to show concerned parties that what we do truly works.

THE FUTURE

Who could have envisioned, 15 years ago, that physicians would be reporting increased survival rates for children weighing 500 g at birth and 23 weeks' gestation? Who could have predicted that the number of children born to adolescent mothers would be at its existing rate? Would it have been possible to predict, 25 years ago, that the number of children born prenatally exposed to drugs would be as high as it is today, or that the number of children born HIV positive would be at its present rate? The answer to each of these questions is clearly, no. No one could have foreseen these events.

As a corollary observation, who could have known in 1973, when legislation was passed mandating services to disabled children 3 to 5 years of age, that in the year 2000 the focus would be on children with special needs from birth and that equal emphasis would be placed on services provided for families? The passage of Public Law 99-457 and all subsequent amendments and early intervention legislation, has literally changed the landscape of efforts to improve the lives of people with disabilities. New technologies, assessment techniques, intervention activities, curricula, personnel preparation methods, and professional standards have emerged. An entire "early intervention" enterprise has materialized.

In education, one factor that remains constant is the probability of change. Families change, professionals change, and child and family needs will continue to change. Effective family-focused early intervention must keep up with changes. This takes dedication, vision, energy, and a commitment to excellence. Many EI professionals, if asked "Can you think of one child/family in your professional career from whom you derive great pleasure as you recall the impact your services had," would be readily able to do so. The pleasure derived from significantly meeting child and family needs cannot be put in monetary terms. Rather, it is the deep sense of satisfaction that EIs receive from a job well done. This text has been conceived to allow more EI professionals to share in the satisfaction of a job well done.

The future of early intervention is bright. It is as full of potential as the eyes of the 2-year-old who desperately wishes to communicate. It is as brimming with hope as the look of the young mother who depends on you, regardless of your anxiety, to help her meet the needs inherent in having a child at significant risk for developmental delay. To provide anything less than the best we can offer to children and parents is to sell them short. The intent of this text is to better equip all EI professionals so that parents, babies, and families might realize their full potential.

REFERENCES

Achenbach, T., Howell, C., Aoki, M., & Rauh, V. (1993). Nine year outcome of the Vermont Intervention Program for Low Birthweight Infants. *Pediatrics, 91*, 45.

Achenbach, T., Phares, V., Howell, C., Rauh, V., & Nurcombe, B. (1990). Seven year outcome of the Vermont Intervention Program for Low Birthweight Infants. *Child Development, 61,* 1672.

Als, H., Lawhon, G., & Duffy, F. (1994). Individualized developmental care for the very low-birth-weight preterm infant: Medical and neurofunctional effects. *Journal of the American Medical Association, 272,* 853–858.

Barba, L., & Walker, C. (1992). Infant definitive care: Developmental care for the hospitalized NICU graduate. *Neonatal Network, 11,* 35.

Barnard, K. (1973). The effect of stimulation on the sleep behavior of the premature infant. *Communicating Nursing Research, 6,* 12.

Barnett, S. (1993). Benefit-cost analysis of preschool education: Findings from a 25-year follow-up. *American Journal of Orthopsychiatry, 63,* 500–508.

Becker, P., Grunwald, P., Moorman, J., & Stuhr, S. (1991). Outcomes of developmentally supportive nursing care for very low birth weight infants. *Nursing Research, 40,* 150–155.

Belsky, J. (1984). The determinants of parenting: A process model. *Child Development, 55,* 83.

Bennett, F., & Guralnick, M. (1992). Promoting development and integration of infants experiencing neonatal intensive care. In K. Haring, D. Lovett, & N. Haring (Eds.), *Integrated life cycle services for persons with disabilities: A theoretical and empirical perspective* (p. 237). New York: Springer-Verlag.

Berrera, M., Kitching, K., Cunningham, C., Douchet, D., & Rosenbaum, P. (1990). A 3-year early home intervention follow-up study with low birthweight infants and their parents. *Topics in Early Childhood Special Education, 10,* 14–28.

Blanchard, Y. (1991). Early intervention and stimulation of the hospitalized preterm infant. *Infants and Young Children, 4,* 76–84.

Bronfenbrenner, U. (1974). *Is early intervention effective?* Washington, DC: Office of Human Development.

Brooks-Gunn, J., Klebanov, P., Liaw, F., & Spiker, D. (1993). Enhancing the development of low-birthweight, premature infants: Changes in cognition and behavior over the first three years. *Child Development, 64,* 736–753.

Bruder, M. (1993). The provision of early intervention and early childhood special education within community early childhood programs: Characteristics of effective service delivery. *Topics in Early Childhood Special Education, 13,* 19–37.

Bryant, D., & Ramey, C. (1987). An analysis of the effectiveness of early intervention programs for environmentally at-risk children. In M. Guralnick & F. Bennett (Eds.), *The effectiveness of early intervention for at-risk and handicapped children* (p. 58). Orlando, FL: Academic Press.

Burns, K., Deddish, R., Burns, W., & Hatcher, R. (1983). Use of oscillating waterbeds and rhythmic sounds for premature infant stimulation. *Developmental Psychology, 19,* 746.

Casto, G., & Mastropieri, M. (1986). The efficacy of early intervention programs: A meta-analysis. *Exceptional Children, 52,* 417.

Committee for Economic Development: Research and Policy Committee. (1987). *Children in need: Investment strategies for the educationally disadvantaged.* New York: Committee for Economic Development.

Dawson, P., Robinson, J., Butterfield, P., van Doornick, W., Gaensbauer, T., & Harmon, R. (1990). Supporting new parents through home visits: Effects on mother-infant interaction. *Topics in Early Childhood Special Education, 10,* 29–44.

Farran, D. (1990). Effects of intervention with disadvantaged and disabled children: A decade review. In S. Meisels and J. Shonkoff (Eds.), *Handbook of early childhood intervention* (p. 211). Cambridge, England: Cambridge University Press.

Fewell, R., & Delwein, P. (1991). Effective early intervention: Results from the model preschool program for children with Down syndrome and other developmental delays. *Topics in Early Childhood Special Education, 11,* 56–68.

Fey, M., & Cleave, P. (1990). Early language intervention. *Seminars in Speech and Language, 11,* 19–33.

Field, T. (1980). Teenage, lower-class, black mothers and their preterm infants: An intervention and developmental follow-up. *Child Development, 51,* 29.

Girolometto, L. (1988). Improving the social-converstional skills of developmentally delayed children: An intervention study. *Journal of Speech and Hearing Disorders, 53,* 156.

Girolometto, L., Greenburg, J., & Manolson, A. (1986). Developing dialogue skills: The Hanen early language training program. *Seminars in Speech and Language, 4,* 367.

Grantham-McGregor, S. (1987). Development of severely malnourished children who received psychosocial stimulation: Six year follow-up. *Pediatrics, 79,* 48.

Grunwald, P., & Becker, P. (1991). Developmental enhancement: Implementing a program for the NICU. *Neonatal Network, 9,* 29.

Guralnick, M. (1988). Efficacy research in early childhood intervention programs. In S. Odom & M. Karnes (Eds.), *Early intervention for infants and children with handicaps: An empirical base* (p. 52). Baltimore: Paul H. Brookes.

Guralnick, M. (1989). Recent developments in early intervention efficacy research: Implications for family involvement in P. L. 99-457. *Topics in Early Childhood Special Education, 9,* 1.

Guralnick, M. (1997). *The effectiveness of early intervention.* Baltimore: Paul H. Brookes.

Guralnick, M., & Bennett, F. (Eds.). (1987). *The effectiveness of early intervention for at-risk and handicapped children.* New York: Academic Press.

Guralnick, M., & Bricker, D. (1987). The effectiveness of early intervention for children with cognitive and general developmental delays. In M. Guralnick & F. Bennett (Eds.), *The effectiveness of early intervention for at-risk and handicapped children* (p. 380). New York: Academic Press.

Harris, S. (1987). Early intervention for children with motor handicaps. In M. Guralnick & F. Bennett (Eds.), *The effectiveness of early intervention for at-risk and handicapped children* (p. 130). New York: Academic Press.

Heincke, C., Beckwith, L., & Thompson, A. (1989). Early intervention in the family system: A framework and review. *Infant Mental Health Journal, 9,* 2.

Heriza, C., & Sweeney, J. (1990). Effects of NICU intervention on preterm infants: Part 1—Implications for neonatal practice. *Infants and Young Children, 2*, 31–40.

Home visiting: A promising early intervention strategy for at-risk families. (1990). Report to the Chairman, Subcommittee on Labor, Health and Human Services, Education, and Related Agencies, Committee on Appropriations, U.S. Senate. Washington DC: General Accounting Office.

Infant Health and Development Program. (1990). Enhancing the outcomes of low birthweight, premature infants: A multisite, randomized trial. *Journal of the American Medical Association, 263*, 30–35.

Innocenti, M., Huh, K., & Boyce, G. (1992). Families of children with disabilities: Normative data and other considerations on parenting stress. *Topics in Early Childhood Special Education, 12*, 403.

Jacobsen, C., Starnes, C., & Gasser, V. (1988). An experimental analysis of the generalization of descriptions and praises for mothers of premature infants. *Human Communication Canada, 12*, 23.

Johnson, D., & Walker, T. (1991). A follow-up evaluation of the Houston Parent-Child Development Center: School performance. *Journal of Early Intervention, 15*, 226.

Katz, V. (1971). Auditory stimulation and developmental behavior of the premature infant. *Nursing Research, 20*, 196.

Korner, A., Kraemer, H., Haffner, M., & Cosper, L. (1975). Effects of waterbed flotation on premature infants: A pilot study. *Pediatrics, 56*, 361.

Kramer, L., & Pierpont, M. (1976). Rocking waterbeds and auditory stimuli to enhance growth of preterm infants. *Journal of Pediatrics, 88*, 297.

Lee, S., & Kahn, J. (1997). Measures of child progress and program effectiveness in early intervention. *Infant Toddler Intervention, 7*, 4.

Leib, S., Benfield, D., & Guidubaldi, J. (1980). Effects of early intervention and stimulation on the preterm infant. *Pediatrics, 66*, 83.

MacDonald, J., & Carroll, J. (1992). A partnership model for communicating with infants at risk. *Infants and Young Children, 4*, 20.

Macfarland-Smith, J., Schuster, J., & Stevens, K. (1993). Using simultaneous prompting to teach expressive object identification to preschoolers with developmental delays. *Journal of Early Intervention, 17*, 50.

Mahoney, G., O'Sullivan, P., & Robinson, C. (1992). The family environments of children with disabilities. *Topics in Early Childhood Special Education, 12*, 386.

Markowitz, J., Hebbeler, K., Larson, J., Cooper, J., & Edmister, P. (1991). Using value-added analysis to examine short-term effects of early intervention. *Journal of Early Intervention, 15*, 337.

Martin, S., Ramey, C., & Ramey, S. (1990). The prevention of intellectual impairment in children of impoverished families: Findings of a randomized trial of educational day care. *American Journal of Public Health, 80*, 844.

McCollum, J. (1991). At the crossroad: Reviewing and rethinking interaction coaching. In K. Marfo (Ed.), *Early intervention in transition: Current perspectives on programs for handicapped children* (p. 90). New York: Praeger.

Meadow-Orlans, K. (1987). An analysis of the effectiveness of early intervention programs for hearing-impaired children. In M. Guralnick & F. Bennett (Eds.), *The effectiveness of early intervention for at-risk and handicapped children* (p. 50). New York: Academic Press.

Meyer, E., Coll, C., & Lester, B. (1994). Family-based intervention improves maternal psychological well-being and feeding interaction of preterm infants. *Pediatrics, 93,* 2.

Meyer, L., & Eichinger, J. (1987). Program evaluation in support of programming development. In L. Goetz, D. Guess, & K. Campbell (Eds.), *Innovative program designs for individuals with dual sensory impairments* (p. 92). Baltimore: Paul H. Brookes.

Miller, C. (1987). *Maternal health and infant survival.* Washington DC: National Center for Clinical Infant Programs.

Olson, M. (1987). Early intervention for children with visual impairments. In M. Guralnick & F. Bennett (Eds.), *The effectiveness of early intervention for at-risk and handicapped children* (p. 130). New York: Academic Press.

Orr, M., Cameron, S., Dobson, L., & Day, D. (1993). Age related changes in stress experienced by families with a child who has developmental delays. *Mental Retardation, 31,* 171.

Parker, S., Zahr, L., Cole, J., & Brecht, M. (1991). Outcome after developmental intervention in the neonatal intensive care unit for mothers of preterm infants with low socioeconomic status. *Journal of Pediatrics, 120,* 780.

Patterson, J., & McCubbin, H. (1983). Chronic illness: Family stress and coping. In H. McCubbin & C. Figley (Eds.), *Stress and the family: Volume II. Coping with catastrophe* (p. 210). New York: Brunner/Mazel.

Peters, M., & Heron, T. (1992). When the best is not good enough: An examination of best practice. *The Journal of Special Education, 26,* 371.

Pinder, G., & Olswang, L. (1995). Development of communicative intent in young children with cerebral palsy: A treatment efficacy study. *Infant-Toddler Intervention, 5,* 51.

Powell, L. (1974). The effect of extra stimulation and maternal involvement on the development of low birthweight infants and on maternal behavior. *Child Development, 45,* 106.

Ramey, C., & Ramey, S. (1992). Effective early intervention. *Mental Retardation, 30,* 337.

Rauh, V. (1988). Minimizing adverse effects of low birthweight: Four-year results of an early intervention program. *Child Development, 59,* 226.

Resnick, M., Armstrong, S., & Carter, R. (1988). Developmental intervention programs for high-risk premature infants: Effects on development and parent-infant interactions. *Journal of Developmental and Behavioral Pediatrics, 9,* 73.

Resnick, M., Eyler, F., Nelson, R., Eitzman, D., & Bucciarelli, R. (1987). Developmental intervention for low birth weight infants: Improved early developmental outcome. *Pediatrics, 80,* 68.

Rice, R. (1977). Neurophysiological development in premature infants following stimulation. *Developmental Psychology, 13,* 69.

Roberts, R. (1991). Early intervention in the home: The interface of policy, programs, and research. *Infants and Young Children, 4,* 33.

Roberts, R., & Wasik, B. (1990). Home visiting programs for families with children birth to three: Results of a national survey. *Journal of Early Intervention, 14*, 274.

Rosenfield, A. G. (1980). Visiting the intensive care nursery. *Child Development, 51*, 939.

Ross, G. (1984). Home intervention for premature infants of low-income families. *American Journal of Orthopsychiatry, 54*, 28.

Rossetti, L. (1990a). *Infant-toddler Assessment: An interdisciplinary approach.* Boston: College-Hill Press.

Sandall, S. (1990). Developmental interventions for biologically at-risk infants at home. *Topics in Early Childhood Special Education, 10*, 1–13.

Segall, M. (1972). Cardiac responsivity to auditory stimulation in premature infants. *Nursing Research, 21*, 15.

Seifer, R., Clark, G., & Sameroff, A. (1991). Positive effects of interaction coaching on infants with developmental disabilities and their mothers. *American Journal of Mental Retardation, 96*, 1.

Shonkoff, J., & Hauser-Cram, P. (1987). Early intervention for disabled infants and their families: A quantitative analysis. *Pediatrics, 80*, 650.

Snyder-McLean, L., & McLean, J. (1987). Effectiveness of early intervention for children with language and communication disorders. In M. Guralnick & F. Bennett (Eds.), *The effectiveness of early intervention for at-risk and handicapped children* (p. 62). New York: Academic Press.

Solomon, R. (1995). Pediatricians and early intervention: Everything you need to know but are too busy to ask. *Infants and Young Children, 7*, 38.

Spiker, D., Ferguson, J., & Brookes-Gunn, J. (1993). Enhancing maternal interactive behavior and child social competence in low birth weight, premature infants. *Child Development, 64*, 754.

Tingey, C. (1989). *Implementing early intervention.* Baltimore: Paul H. Brookes.

VandenBerg, K. (1996). Developmental care, is it working? *Neonatal Network, 15*, 1.

Westrup, B., Klebeg, A., & Hugo, L. (1999). A randomized, controlled trial to evaluate the effects of the newborn individualized developmental care and assessment program in a Swedish setting. *Pediatrics, 105*, 1.

White, J., & Labarba, R. (1976). The effects of tactile and kinesthetic stimulation on neonatal development in the premature infant. *Developmental Psychobiology, 9*, 569.

Wilson, L., Passero, V., & King, W. (1994). An educational program for neonatal intensive care unit developmental care. *Neonatal Network, 13*, 27.

Index

A

Abnormal-abnormal development, 106
Abnormal-normal development, 106
Action-oriented activities, 240–241
Activity, assessment of, 93–94
Adjustment difficulties, parental, 70–72
Adolescent mothers, 25–28, 48–49
    common consequences of early childbearing, 26
Adult goals to facilitate communication, 233
AEPS Measurement for Birth to Three Years, 161–162
African American infants, infant mortality rates of, 27
Aggressive touch, 188
AIDS, pediatric, 32–33
Altered behavior responses in ill infants, 59
Apnea, 23–24
Arena assessment, 120, 122–124
Assessing prelinguistic and early linguistic behaviors in developmentally
        young children, 163
Assessment of socio-communicative skills in infants and toddlers, causation
        models of, 91–93
    current model, 92–93
    historical model, 91–92
    criterion-referenced tests (CRTs), 96–102
        inferences, 102
        samples of behavior, 100–102
    definition of assessment, 93–96
        as activity, 93–94
        medical records report, 94–95
        other EI reports, 95
        parental data, 94
        test results, 95–96
    diagnosis versus assessment, 90–91
    norm-referenced tests, 96–99
        limitations of, 96–99

E

K

L

M

N